Physiotherapy for People with Learning Difficulties

Physiotherapy for People with Learning Difficulties

PATRICIA ODUNMBAKU AUTY

Woodhead-Faulkner

NEW YORK LONDON TORONTO
SYDNEY TOKYO SINGAPORE

Published by Woodhead-Faulkner (Publishers) Limited,
Simon & Schuster International Group,
Fitzwilliam House, 32 Trumpington Street,
Cambridge CB2 1QY, England

First published 1991

© Woodhead-Faulkner (Publishers) Limited, 1991

British Library Cataloguing in Publication Data

Auty, Patricia Odunmbaku
  Physiotherapy for people with learning difficulties.
  I. Title
  615.82

  ISBN 0–85941–663–1

Designed by Geoff Green
Typeset by The Midlands Book Typesetting Co., Loughborough
Printed in Great Britain by BPCC Wheatons Ltd., Exeter

To Karen, Jackie and David,
three clients who taught me

Contents

Acknowledgements

I would like to thank Olive Forshaw, Martin Hutchinson, Pamela Eaton, Sarah Bruce and Gill Howgego for their assistance in the preparation of this book. I would also like to thank my husband Bernard and my daughter Clarefrances for their patience and encouragement, and Pat Layzell without whom this book would not have been written.

Introduction

People with learning difficulties have always been present in society. They have been treated in a variety of ways depending on the culture or beliefs of their society. This treatment ranged from being cast out by the tribe or community, being considered objects of amusement, being thought of as 'close to God' for their simplicity, to euthanasia. They have been called by many names over the years: morons, retards, idiots, lunatics and feeble-minded – all labels which have been devaluing and demeaning.

The terminology in this service is changing rapidly and there has been much debate about the appropriateness of the terms used and the devaluing and dehumanising connotations such labels have. This debate will continue for some time to come as alternative titles are discussed – whether it be 'intellectually impaired people', or 'people with an intellectual disability' or another term.

In the 1980s people with learning difficulties were categorised as having a 'mental handicap'. This term is no longer in favour because of the common confusion of mental handicap and mental illness. The term 'learning difficulties' has been chosen by British people themselves as a more appropriate description if one is required. Thus in this text the term used will be 'people with learning difficulties'. People with a learning difficulty need to learn new skills in an environment which aids their ability to learn and at a pace which is tailored to their individual needs.

It is the belief that people with learning difficulties can and do learn, and that they should be given every opportunity to fulfil their potential, that has prompted this book. One needs to have expectations of people with learning difficulties so that they in turn will have belief in and expectations for and of themselves. Physiotherapists with this appreciation and commitment can make a significant contribution to the quality of life of people with learning difficulties.

The articles quoted in this book must be seen in historical context. Their terminology will help to show the attitudes and approaches then prevalent. The term 'client' denotes both child and adult in this book.

Chapter 1

Physiotherapy and social role valorisation

Introduction

There are many definitions of 'social role valorisation'. In 1972 Wolf Wolfensberger defined it as 'the utilization of cultural valued means in order to establish and/or maintain personal behaviour, experiences and characteristics that are culturally normative or valued'. This principle was restated by John O'Brien and Alan Tyne (1981) as 'the use of means which are valued in our society in order to develop and support personal behaviour, experiences and characteristics which are likewise valued'. A simplified version of this is to grant people with learning difficulties the same rights as the rest of the population, to give them support when required and to afford them the same dignity, communication and understanding that we require for ourselves.

Where and how should people with learning difficulties live? What rights do they have? What choices and decisions are they party to? Until recently, most of them lived within self-sufficient institutions. It is normal to live in the community with one's family or friends. It is normal to have personal possessions and a choice in the decisions affecting one's life and lifestyle. All the basic rights of human beings should be given to everyone – this is what the principle of normalisation is about.

It was evident that there was a need for such a principle to be stated in order to change attitudes and services for people with learning difficulties when institutions and their routines became known to the general population. It is a statement of principle that everyone has the same rights to a valued lifestyle and quality of life. In 1971 the United Nations published 'The declaration of the rights of the mentally retarded person', which was a step forward in highlighting the needs of people with learning difficulties.

The term 'normalisation' was at times misunderstood – normalisation is not trying to 'normalise' a person but bringing about a more normal lifestyle for each person, with support being provided as and when necessary. In an article in 1983 Wolfensberger proposed to change the name to prevent misunderstanding. Since 'the highest goal of the principle of normalisation was to be the establishment, enhancement or defence of the social role/s of the person or group via the enhancement of people's social images and personal competences', the term 'social role valorisation' (SRV) became accepted.

There were many people who were instrumental in bringing this concept to the institutions and services throughout the world. Bank Mikkelsen, head of the Danish Mental Retardation Service, had the concept written into Danish law for the service to the mentally handicapped. Bengt Nirje, then Executive Director of the Swedish Association of Retarded Children, first wrote about 'normalisation' in the late 1960s (Nirje 1970). Wolf Wolfensberger continued with this concept in America, writing many books and articles on the subject. With Linda Glenn he developed a way of measuring the application of this philosophy to the human service, and published it in a book called *Program Analysis of Service Systems* ('PASS') (Wolfensberger and Glenn 1973).

PASS sets a standard by which the service provided for people with learning difficulties can be measured and judged. Factors such as the physical setting are rated – the building, the facilities available, the activities provided within, their appropriateness in terms of the age of the people concerned, the level of integration into a community setting, how people are grouped for various activities, what opportunities there are to mix with non-handicapped people, and so on. Social integration can be affected by the names of the locations in which the services for people with learning difficulties are situated: calling a road Asylum Road is an obvious example. There are many aspects of social role valorisation, and PASS provides instructions for the measurement of each one.

It is important to understand why the philosophy of social

role valorisation has had such an effect on people with learning difficulties. It has been the basis not only for community care but also for changing attitudes, changing services and, most important of all, changing the lives of people with learning difficulties. They are now seen as people who should have opportunities to learn, live and socialise, and who have the same right to a valued lifestyle as the rest of us. It is difficult to appreciate the significance of social role valorisation without an understanding of the history and treatment of people with learning difficulties before the concept was accepted.

Pre-industrial revolution

Attitudes towards children born outside the expected physical or mental norm varied according to the community, culture, beliefs, superstitions or traditions of the society they were born into. The mortality rate was high, but those who lived and who were accepted into their family units were cared for as members of the family. In village communities the lifestyle was slower and simpler. The child would learn simple tasks required within the community and therefore could take part in the life of his or her society. Villages were small and people knew each other. As those with learning difficulties grew up, they were generally protected and cared for, safe within their community and valued as contributing members. Those who were not accepted were abandoned to their fate.

Industrial revolution

The industrial revolution changed many people's lifestyles. People migrated to the industrial centres and began working in the new factories that were mushrooming throughout the country. Life became stressful and work in the factories became complex. People with learning difficulties found this environment more hostile. They were less able to learn and adapt to the quickened pace of life, while the caring village community was lost and community support decreased as the population struggled to make a living. Families were less able to cope with their handicapped members and many were abandoned on to the streets.

New attitudes were changing society, and people became less and less tolerant of those who could not conform to society's rigid standards or keep up with the pace of ordinary life. It became shameful to have a child with learning difficulties, and some adults were often hidden away because of the shame. Sadly, some believed that a handicap in the family was retribution for past deeds.

Fear and ignorance lead to a belief that 'mentally handicapped' people had to be put out of sight. The supposed link between those diagnosed as 'mental defectives' and social problems such as criminality and promiscuity contributed significantly to the call for the segregation of people with learning difficulties. It was believed that allowing the 'defective and incompetent' to bear children would lead to the downfall of the human race.

The Victorian solution was to build large independent communities in rural areas for the long-term care, protection and training of the 'feeble-minded'. Until that time people with learning difficulties were not seen as a distinctive group either in law or in institutional establishments. A study of American asylums in 1820–30 found separate institutions for lunatics and paupers but not for 'idiots', as was the current terminology. This was true of most countries so the exact number of people with learning difficulties was not known. The Victorians built institutions such as the Asylum for Idiots at Park House, Highgate in 1847 and Starcross Asylum in Essex in 1846, to name but two. Many Victorians were in favour of such institutions for charitable reasons while others supported segregation in order to prevent the 'contamination' of society. The movement for the systematic social protection and control of the 'feeble-minded' dates back to the mid-nineteenth century, with the establishment of state and private institutions for the long-term care, protection and treatment of people with learning difficulties in Britain, continental Europe and the USA.

In 1881 a census of 'idiots' in public institutions identified 29,452 people of whom only 3 per cent were in special 'idiot' asylums. By 1914, six special institutions had been built housing 2,040 'idiots'. These were small by 1950 standards, when one institution could be home to 2,000 people. In the book *Community Care and the Mentally Handicapped*, Sam Ayer and Andy Alaszewski show that the provision of places for the 'mental defectives' almost doubled from 1931 when there was a total of 28,234 places to 1939 when the number of places increased to 46,054. In 1961 there were 61,000 people living in institutions. The highest figure reached was 64,000 (Bone et al., 1972). These institutions were self-contained and incorporated their own churches, shops, workshops and even farms. Some enlightened establishments worked to teach the 'inmates' a trade or useful occupation and many of them were involved in helping around the establishment in which they lived. Some worked in the laundry room, repaired shoes or helped in the kitchens, and in this way they felt valued and useful. Their work also contributed significantly to the care of the severely handicapped since staff were always in short supply.

The original concept of care training and protection was admirable according to the precepts of the day. However, not all establishments provided such activities and many people walked aimlessly around large soulless corridors for most of the time. In the early days, uniforms were provided and strict segregation of the sexes was enforced. Unfortunately, some of these institutions were used as a dumping ground for people who had offended against the moral code of the day: for example, a girl having a child out of wedlock was often put with her child into an institution to prevent them shaming the family. Many of these unfortunate people lived their whole lives within the confines of the institutions – a sad waste of life.

Many physically handicapped and non-verbal-communicating people were misdiagnosed and put into institutions for the 'feeble-minded' where they lived silent lives within large groups of people. The distress caused to them is immeasurable. Privacy was a rare commodity; it was difficult to allow people the time to go to the bathroom on their own when they lived in a dormitory with so many others and when there were so few staff to supervise them. It was easier for the staff to monitor people if they all went to the bathroom at the same time, which created a lack of dignity and a loss of personal awareness and individualism. Although this practice was not always condoned by the staff in the institutions, it was the only way that the few staff on a large ward could watch over and protect their charges. Unfortunately, over time the practice became habitual and unquestioned, and it contributed to a loss of a valued lifestyle for the people who lived there. Institutional clothing, little contact with the outside world and no personal possessions contributed to poor self-image and self-worth.

In England the County Asylums and Madhouse Act required regular inspections by the Metropolitan Commissioners, who drew the public's attention to the poor conditions within some asylums. The Lunatics Act 1845 extended the power of the Commissioners to inspect all asylums and 'madhouses' throughout the country. There were some scandals of malpractice and abuse which horrified the public, and their reaction led to much needed reforms. One such scandal was the fire at York Asylum in 1813. In more recent times the conditions for the patients at Ely Hospital in Cardiff caused an outcry and created pressure for reform in 1969.

It was a commonly held belief until recent times that parents should be advised to put a child with a learning difficulty into an institution where he or she could be cared for. Many people were put into institutions by caring parents who were told by their physician that they should put the children away and forget them; they would not learn and would never be able to live within society, and so contact with the outside world was actively discouraged. Other devoted families continued to visit their children for many years. People in institutions became demotivated and dependent as they were allowed to do very little for themselves.

The twentieth century

In an article called 'Ward 99' in the *Nursing Times*, John Brown (1972) gives a vivid description of a day in the life of forty-seven severely 'mentally retarded handicapped males':

> Nothing prepares the new (and often untrained) member of staff for the conditions on Ward 99. It is possible to get used to distressing sights and even to the continual deafening clamour which assails the ears. Even the regular staff did not get used to the smell, and all except one (who boasted of the fact) occasionally had to wear surgical masks when changing incontinent patients – a task which was to dominate the day's routine.

In an article in *New Society* Michael Bury (1974) describes the daily routine of those with 'severe sub-normality', and in 'The back ward syndrome', Peter Williams *et al.* (1975) continue a description of the full impact of Ward 99 and its

> low grade mentally handicapped men, some in wheel-chairs, some moving painfully and clumsily, some gazing vacantly into space, some repeating ritual gestures with curious intensity; the sound of a deafening and meaningless clamour which never abates, even at mealtimes; the touch of many hands, all seeking human contact, all demanding; and the smell of double incontinence so strong that it became a taste in the mouth, and deadens the appetite.

These articles give an understanding of the attitudes of the time, the people in the institutions and the expectations of the staff for the patients in their care. It is understandable that many people felt there was a need for change.

The names of these closed communities changed from asylums, places of refuge for lunatics (no distinction being drawn in those days between mentally ill and mentally handicapped people), to hospitals – with all their medical connotations. The foundations of the present services were laid in the 1920s and 1930s. The public authority had statutory responsibilities for the services provided for people with learning difficulties. However, the underlying principles were different from those observed today.

Until 1948 local authorities were responsible for all aspects of care for the 'mentally handicapped'. They provided 'supervision' for the inmates of the institutions. The superintendent was usually a doctor, and the staff were called attendants.

The National Health Service in 1948 took over responsibility for the institutions when they became hospitals and the inmates became patients, encouraging the belief that learning difficulty was an illness which involved doctors and psychiatrists. Thus the medical model of care was established. More recently, attitudes changed and mental handicap was seen not as an illness but as a social problem of learning. 'Patient' was dropped in favour of 'client' or 'user of the service', and efforts were made to give hospitals a more homely environment, to adopt the philosophy of social role valorisation and to improve attitudes.

Over the years in England there were many changes within the institutions – some good, some bad – but many institutions provided occupations and activities for the people living within their walls and tried to make life as rewarding and interesting as possible. In 1959 the Mental Handicap Act laid down the early foundations for change. After this various documents repeatedly advocated more attention to research into active therapy and improving the effectiveness of hospital services for the 'subnormal'. Smaller hospitals were also advocated, but this was easier said than done. For example, in 1968 Leavesden Hospital in Hertfordshire had 1,300 people living there and in 1989 there were still 800 residents.

In 1960 Northgate Hospital in Morpeth, Northumberland, began working for a multi-disciplinary approach so that the adults and children in the hospital had continuous treatment. Physiotherapists visited the centre for three sessions a week, handing on their skills to the nurses who carried out the treatment programmes arranged for the clients. This was a new concept at the time, in line with government policy.

Changing old accepted practice was daunting; changing the environment was costly; but changing attitudes and expectations was the most difficult. Thomas Pilkington, writing in the *British Hospital Journal and Social Services Review*, inferred that the 'biggest obstacle to change was the attitudes of staff'. He also wrote that it was clear that hospitals could not provide comprehensive care for all the 'retarded'. 'It was equally clear local government could not cope with the problems of providing training centres and hostels.' He further stated that 'there was a limited place for the latter and the bulk of long term support must come from the community' (Pilkington, 1967).

In 1968 nurses were coping with the recommendations of the Salmon Report. A new training student syllabus was implemented to improve the conditions and status of the nurses in this speciality. It was in December 1969 that the Secretary of State, Richard Crossman, became enraged about the indignities heaped upon the men and women who lived in hospitals for the mentally handicapped. After visiting many of these institutions, he realised that money alone would not solve the problem. Staff needed the opportunity to learn new skills and new attitudes, and the time to develop their existing skills and knowledge. Crossman saw that training was essential to the future. Training Project Officers were appointed to help organise broad discussions with a view to improving staff training and providing the best possible care for the mentally handicapped. This care had to go hand in hand with the programmes of physical improvement if these were to have their maximum effect (remedial gymnasts and physiotherapists have helped to fulfil this objective).

Much interest and discussion followed this statement, and many articles were written at the time, some decrying the new atitudes and some supporting them. Discussions continue even now regarding the need for change. It was this desire to change attitudes towards the mentally handicapped, and the quality of life of people living away from society, that created the philosophy of normalisation.

Care in the community

Although government policy had since 1959 urged a move towards a community-based service, people were still being admitted for long-term care during the 1960s. However, in 1970 the inadequacy of hospital provision was publicly acknowledged and hospitals reduced the number of people on their wards. This was mainly done through discontinuing long-term admission of children and through a reduction in beds following the natural demise of the elderly hospital population.

'Better services for the mentally handicapped' (HMSO, 1971) advocated returning patients to the community. This caused considerable concern to the people responsible for those with a mental handicap, since they felt that the community would be a hostile environment for them. Robert O'Toole, writing in the British Hospital Journal and Social Services Review, stated the premiss 'that the mentally handicapped have as much right to choice and fulfilment within society as the rest of us'. His question was 'Have they also as much right to lack of choice and frustration as the rest of us?'(O'Toole, 1972).

As the philosophy of social role valorisation became more understood and accepted, gradual changes were made within hospitals. New smaller hospitals were built, and small villa-style houses aimed at creating a more village-like atmosphere. Fieldhead Hospital, Wakefield, which opened in 1973, was built to this model. There was accommodation for eighty children, with suitable play rooms and sandpits, and even pet shelters were built so that children could have pets. This represents a considerable change of attitude.

In 1976 the Development Team came into existence, now called the National Team for Mentally Handicapped People. It is a multi-disciplinary group of professionals who have expertise in planning developmental and operational issues and can advise and assist health authorities, voluntary organisations and social services on the resettlement of clients into the community.

In 1979 an initiative was started to improve the lives of people with learning difficulties. The goal was to see mentally handicapped people in the mainstream of life, living in ordinary houses in ordinary streets, with the same range of choice as any citizen, and mixing as equals with the others, and mostly not handicapped members of the community.

To develop this initiative each health authority set about planning and providing different models of care within its district. There was also an exchange of ideas and expertise between countries, learning from each other and helping to establish a suitable model. Some built small core and cluster-type villages; others provided a comprehensive range of educational, residential and vocational services for their people within the community. One such establishment was the Eastern Nebraska Community Office of Retardation ('ENCOR'), which provided services in the area where its people and their families lived. They commissioned multi-disciplinary professionals to provide the appropriate services to clients.

Darenth Park Hospital in Kent was the first English hospital to close and establish community care. It began as Darenth School for five hundred children in 1878, and ten years later there were a thousand adults and children there. By 1911 it was called Darenth Industrial Training Colony and in 1936 it was renamed Darenth Park Hospital. It was run by the London County Council until the National Health Service became responsible for it in 1948. Although children were not admitted after 1934, short-term admittance started in 1952, and in 1954 long-term admittance began again because of local demand. The hospital had a wide catchment area including London, but it also had some people from the rest of the country. It was a large isolated hospital housing about a thousand people in 1979.

A paper called 'Closing a Hospital: The Darenth Park project' by Nancy Korman and Howard Glennerster detailed the planning required. This was followed by a book called *Hospital Closure*, which gives a comprehensive account of the planning, organisation and evaluation of such a major task (Korman and Glennerster, 1990).

As the people living at Darenth Park came from many places in the south-east of England, it was necessary to contact their districts of origin so that the latter would resume responsibility for their clients and resettle them. This was an enormous undertaking. Each district decided on the model of care it wished to provide and set up services accordingly. Darenth Park was replaced by a network of community homes, hostels and day centres mainly in the south-east of England. Some districts entered into a consortium of housing associations and charitable institutions to buy and manage houses for their clients to live in.

The necessary services were provided in most cases by the health authority through community and multi-disciplinary mentally handicapped teams set up in the area. Some districts bought land and built houses for seventy or eighty people around a day centre which also housed the therapists involved with providing a service for those clients. Others built resource centres with a hydrotherapy pool, day centre, physiotherapy unit and play group on site, for clients living in the community. There were many housing schemes, from fifteen young men living in a group home, to three people sharing a house, to a client living in his or her own home and supported by volunteers, to people living independently. Whichever model was chosen, it took a number of years to complete the transition from institutional care to district-based community care.

Houses were only a small part of the planning. The support system and the level of care required to enable a client to live in the community and have the opportunity for growth and learning also required considerable finance and thought. There are versions of these models in different countries throughout Europe.

The transition from institutional care to care in the community has been a difficult and in some cases traumatic time for clients and established staff within hospitals as all face a new and uncertain future. There has been fear of the unknown and genuine concern that the community would be unaccepting of people coming from institutions – as well as anxiety that those who have been institutionalised for forty or fifty years will not be able to live outside a hospital. With the correct support and environment, however, all these fears have proved groundless.

The provision of community-based services has been guided by the philosophy of social role valorisation, which has not only influenced the thinking and planning of the services, but also affected the lives of the users. However, giving people with learning difficulties the opportunity for growth and learning requires considerable finance and planning. Community care is not a cheap option.

The service for learning difficulties provided in the community varies considerably from district to district. Some have a more formal, organised team consisting of administrator, support manager, speech therapist, physiotherapist, occupational therapist and social worker, sometimes headed by a patch manager. Others have a less formal structure consisting of a social worker, nurse and support worker, who refer clients to therapists in the service when necessary. Unfortunately, some districts have only a single physiotherapist trying to provide a service to all the clients in the community. Physiotherapists are in short supply in this undervalued area. Sometimes there are only one or two therapists working from an Acute Unit who have an interest in this client group.

Whatever service is provided to the users, it is based around their individual needs and a philosophy of social role valorisation which can be evaluated by PASS. With the changes in the Health Service and both the White Paper 'Working for patients' and the Griffiths Report of 1988 there will be more changes to the services to be provided for clients living within the community (HMSO, 1988, 1989). From 1 April 1991, when changes recommended in the White Paper became reality, contracts for the delivery of services to people with learning difficulties were made. This may affect how the service will be delivered.

Will the generic service become solely responsible for everyone living in the community, including people with learning difficulties? Will there be a need for a specialist service which could be bought in by the commissioning authority provided by social services, or will there still be a need for the health authority to provide for those with multiple needs?

References

Alaszewski, A. (1986) *Institutional Care and Mental Handicap*, London: Croom Helm.

Bone, M., Spain, B. and Fox, M. (1972) *Plans and Provision for Mental Handicap*, London: Allen & Unwin.

Brown, J. (1972) 'Ward 99', *Nursing Times*, February.

Bury, M. (1974) 'Life on Yellow Ward', New *Society*, May.

HMSO (1971) 'Better services for the mentally handicapped', London: HMSO.

HMSO (1988) *Community Care: An agenda for action* (Griffiths Report), London: HMSO, ref. 0113211309.

HMSO (1989) 'Working for patients. The Health Service: caring for the 1990s', White Paper, London: HMSO, Cm555.

Korman, K. and Glennerster, H. (1990) *Hospital Closure: A political and economic study*, Milton Keynes: Open University Press.

Nirje, B. (1970) 'The normalization principle: implications and comments', *Journal of Mental Subnormality*, vol. 16, pp. 62–70.

O'Brien, John (1981) *Principles of Normalisation: A foundation for effective services*, London: Campaign for People with Mental Handicap. Adapted for CMH by A. Tyne.

O'Toole, R. (1972) 'New deal for mentally handicapped', *British Hospital Journal and Social Service Review*, 29 July.

Pilkington, T. (1967) 'The changing subnormality hospital', *British Hospital Journal and Social Service Review*, 3 February.

United Nations (1971) 'Declaration of the rights of mentally retarded persons', resolution adopted by the General Assembly of the United Nations, 3rd committee (A/8588) 2856, 2027th plenary meeting, December.

Williams, P., Brown, J. and Jones, K. (1975) 'The back ward syndrome', New *Society*, 3 July.

Wolfensberger, W. (1972) *The Principle of Normalisation in Human Services*, Toronto: National Institute on Mental Retardation.

Wolfensberger, W. and Glenn, L. (1973) *Program Analysis of Service Systems (PASS): A method for the quantitative evaluation of human services*, Field Manual, Toronto: National Institute on Mental Retardation.

Wolfensberger, W. (1983) 'Mental retardation', *American Association on Mental Deficiency*, vol. 21, no. 6, pp. 234–9.

Chapter 2

Learning difficulties

Introduction

Finding a satisfactory definition of 'learning difficulties' has proved very difficult. There are many historical descriptions which were acceptable in their day but would not now be the correct or acceptable terminology. Those with learning difficulties are a heterogeneous collection of people with a wide range of genetic, environmental, sensory and physical handicaps, each of which can limit their opportunities and abilities. People who have learning difficulties learn slowly to adjust to other people's perceptions of behaviour, living models and attitudes. However, they require varying levels of assistance to do so.

The definition of 'mental handicap' in the Mental Health Act 1987 does not do justice to the clients whose main impairment is the inability to adapt easily to the environment and to the demands of daily life. Another of the many terms used is 'mental retardation', which is the standard terminology in the USA and Canada.

Physiotherapists are concerned with enabling clients to increase their functions and independence, and they do this by responding to the needs of the client. A diagnosis is not necessary, since the careful assessment of the client's referred needs provides all the information required to plan a programme for that client. In many cases the diagnosis is not known. While it might be interesting to know the cause, it is not essential; we are not, nor should we be, in a medical model attitude of care.

Although there are numerous medical and environmental conditions which contribute to the development of learning disability, and these can occur before, during or after birth, learning difficulty is not an illness and therefore cannot be 'cured'. However, the development of people with learning difficulties can be improved by education, training and social care.

The clinical causes of learning difficulty are many and can be categorised as follows:

1. Chromosomal abnormalities.
2. Metabolic disorders.
3. Environmental factors.

Chromosomal abnormalities

The cells' nuclei hold the hereditary information of the individual in their rod-shaped chromosomes. There are 46 chromosomes, of which 44 are the same in the male and female (these are called autosomes). The remaining two chromosomes determine the sex of the individual and are XX in the female and XY in the male. Chromosomes carry the genes which, acting either individually or in combination with others, determine a person's physical and mental characteristics.

There are many chromosomal abnormalities. These include the possession of extra chromosomes, the absence of chromosomes, additional chromosome materials and chromosome alterations. The presence of an extra chromosome is known as trisomy.

Down's syndrome (Trisomy 21)

This condition was first described by John Langdon-Down in 1866 and has been one of the most common chromosome abnormalities. It consists of a group of characteristics which occur when a baby is born with 47 chromosomes rather than 46. The extra chromosome is at pair 21, producing an autosomal trisomy. This leads to slow learning and physical characteristics which include mongoloid features, poor muscle tone, cardiac abnormalities and, particularly in children, chest infections. Down's syndrome can be detected *in utero* by amniocentesis test or chorion biopsy.

Edward's syndrome (Trisomy 17–18)

This condition is the second most common autosomal abnormality. The extra chromosome is at pair 18. Clients may have abnormalities in muscle tone which can vary from hypertonia to hypotonia. They usually have small delicate facial features with an elongation of the skull and receding chin. 'Rocker bottom' feet, limited hip movement and spasticity can all be present.

Cri du chat

There may be deletions of part of a chromosome, which can result in the loss of genetic material from either the short or the long arms of one of the autosomal pairs. Cri du chat is caused by partial deletion of the short arm of one of the chromosomes at pair 5. It is so named because of the cat-like cry of the baby. Children may be born with low birth weight and their subsequent growth may be retarded. The condition gives rise to multiple deformities including microcephaly. It affects females more than males and produces severe learning difficulties.

Lawrence Moon Biedl syndrome

This is inherited in an autosomal recessive gene. It is characterised by obesity, retinal degeneration and underdevelopment of the genitalia. Where the degree of learning difficulty is severe there may also be associated hearing loss and epilepsy.

Sturge–Webber syndrome

This is a disorder characterised by a cutaneous haemangiomata of the face (port-wine-coloured nevus). Malformation of the meninges, frequent cerebral calcification, epilepsy and learning difficulties of varying degrees occur. Less frequent findings are hemiparesis and glaucoma. The condition usually appears sporadically without familial incidents.

Rett's syndrome

This is a rare disorder which only affects girls. Apparently normal development up to nine months is followed by regression of behaviour and skills. There is usually a reduction in the rate of head growth and a loss of manipulative ability. Habitual hand-wringing movements occur and emotional behaviour changes as the child becomes withdrawn and anxious. Autistic features develop, and spasticity of the limbs increases with age. If walking is achieved, it is with a wide-legged gait to assist their unsteady balance. Spinal curvature may develop in adolescence, and this is sometimes surgically corrected. Epilepsy is a common feature of the disease.

Metabolic disorders

Phenylketonuria syndrome

This is a disorder of protein metabolism, which if untreated results in profound learning difficulties. The child is normal at birth but the process of intellectual damage occurs as the new-born child ingests protein. An autosomal recessive gene causes a deficiency of the enzymes normally present in the liver to convert phenylalanine to tyrosine. This results in raised levels of phenylalanine in the blood, which is toxic to the developing brain and results in brain damage. It is a preventable disorder which can be treated by placing the new-born child on a low phenylalanine diet.

Galactosaemia syndrome

This is a disorder of carbohydrate metabolism characterised by failure to thrive, enlargement of the liver and spleen, development of cataract, and learning difficulties for those who are not diagnosed and treated. An autosomal recessive gene causes an absence or deficiency of the enzymes necessary for conversion of galactose. Treatment is achieved by restricting galactose in the diet. The result will be normal body function and a lessening or prevention of learning difficulties.

Tay–Sachs disease

This is a condition of abnormal storage of lipid (fat) material in tissues, which leads to tissue degeneration. It is an autosomal recessive gene defect where there is a deficiency of an enzyme essential for normal lipid metabolism. It is a disease which occurs almost exclusively among the Ashkenazy Jews, now predominantly within urban communities in the USA.

Microcephaly

This is a generic term which refers to an abnormally small brain and skull. It can be of genetic or non-genetic origin. In the genetic form it can be inherited in a simple autosomal recessive gene; the non-genetic or environmental form is secondary to various disease processes which arrest brain development. Microcephaly presents as a narrow head and receding forehead with small cranium and flattened occiput, which gives the head a conical appearance. This becomes more noticeable as the child grows, although the entire body is dwarfed and underweight. Children with microcephaly are often hypertonic, and about a third of them have seizures and profound learning difficulties.

In most countries microcephaly due to autosomal recessive gene transmission is rare, but where consanguineous unions are common it may occur in substantial numbers. Research has shown this in certain south Indian communities. Similar conditions can be found in isolated communities or cultural, religious or social enclaves.

Environmental factors

Environmental factors include acute or chronic lack of oxygen, childhood or maternal infections, trauma, maternal–foetal incapability, tetrogenic substances, and sensory and social deprivation.

Anoxia

Lack of oxygen even for brief periods can cause damage to the developing brain. This can result in a complex group of disorders of movement and posture.

Cerebral palsy
This condition, first described by J. Little in 1853, means a paralysis of cerebral origin. It can also be associated with learning difficulty depending on the area of brain damage. From birth infants begin to comprehend spacial relations by moving their bodies, and they obtain visual, kinaesthetic, tactile and proprioceptive feedback in this way. With severe cerebral palsy the child may not be able to initiate movement, so experience of spacial awareness, etc. will be limited and underdeveloped. There are a variety of motor problems, weakness, paralysis, incoordination, involuntary or jerky movements, imbalance and variability of muscle tone.

The brain lesion which is responsible for spasticity is in the pyramidal tract, the motor pathways that descend from the cortex and control voluntary muscle. Depending on the area of the cortex involved, it can affect one side of the body, resulting in hemiplegia; both legs more than the arms, resulting in diplegia; or all four limbs, resulting in quadriplegia.

Dyskinetic cerebral palsy
This condition is characterised by impairment of motion by uncontrolled, purposeless movements which disappear during sleep. There are variations in muscle tone from flaccidity to hypertonisity. The lesion is in the basal ganglia, which affects the extra pyramidal motor tracks. The most common type known is athetoid cerebral palsy.

Ataxia cerebral palsy
This is a more rare form which results in poor balance, requiring a wide base to assist in standing or walking. The lesion is in the cerebellum or its pathways.

Infections

Rubella (German or three-day measles)
This is a common communicable disease of childhood. If contracted in early pregnancy it may cause severe congenital abnormalities in the newborn infant. It presents with a variety of sensory problems from deafness and blindness to associated problems

of physical handicap. Active immunisation of children and nonpregnant, post-pubertal females who have been shown to have a negative haemagglutination inhibition test and who will not be pregnant for at least three months is encouraged in the USA. European countries tend to immunise all girls of twelve years.

Toxoplasmosis
Toxoplasmosis in the pregnant woman can cause problems in the developing embryo, such as microcephaly and motor dysfunction. The infection is caused by an organism called *Toxoplasma gondii.*

Meningitis
Meningitis is a systemic infection of the menginges of the brain. The damage varies proportionately with the severity of the infection.

Trauma

Accidental injury
Car accidents causing severe brain damage can result in hemiplegia, epilepsy and learning difficulties which may be slight but may be associated with behavioural and personality changes which limit the person's learning potential.

Non-accidental injury
Maternal battering and the battered-baby syndrome can lead to learning difficulties and other physical disabling conditions.

Maternal–foetal incompatibility

Rhesus factor
When a Rhesus negative mother is pregnant with a Rhesus positive child, the first child is usually unharmed but in subsequent pregnancies antibodies which have developed during the first pregnancy can damage the red blood cells. This causes concentration of bile pigments which affect the basal ganglia and auditory centres in the child. Learning difficulties and associated physical disabilities such as spasticity and athetoid movements may also be present.

Tetrogenic agents

Tetrogenic agents can cause a number of physical problems from ataxia to paralysis and intellectual impairment.

Alcohol
Severe alcoholism of the mother during pregnancy can cause intellectual impairment, poor foetal growth and neurodevelopmental problems. When monitored in the USA this was seen as an important cause of learning difficulties.

Drugs
Drugs taken during a pregnancy can affect the foetus both physically (as in the case of thalidomide) and intellectually. Insulin used to treat maternal diabetes mellitus may induce foetal hypoglycaemia, which may be severe enough to cause brain damage and learning difficulties. Other drugs have been shown to cause intellectual impairment. Drugs used in the treatment of epilepsy, for example, can affect the foetus.

Smoking
Smoking during pregnancy can cause foetal underdevelopment, possibly by reducing the placental blood flow, causing anoxia.

Sensory and social factors

Disabilities of sight, hearing, taste or smell interrupt the child's correct interpretation of the environment. This can be overcome, but it is more difficult when someone also has a learning difficulty since it further delays development. Clients deprived of stimulation or social interaction may become withdrawn, present with autistic tendencies and fail to achieve their full potential.

Epilepsy

Epilepsy can be part of many of the above conditions. There are recurrent attacks associated with altered states of consciousness and usually a succession of tonic or clonic muscle spasms. These attacks, seizures, fits or convulsions may also include abnormal sensory experiences and disturbed behaviour. Epilepsy may be found in isolated incidences in infants with hyperthermia and never recur.

The electrical activity of the brain can be recorded using an electroencephalograph (EEG). From the recorded trace, information can be obtained on the form or type of epilepsy.

The seizures can be categorised as follows.

Grand mal
In grand mal the client can fall to the ground, lose consciousness and become rigid. He or she may then have convulsive movements lasting a few minutes. If many grand mal seizures follow successively without the client regaining consciousness *status epilepticus* can occur.

Petit mal
In petit mal attacks consist of brief interruptions of consciousness ranging from a few seconds to the blink of an eye. This is more common in childhood.

There are many people whose learning difficulty entails no more than slow and restricted development, uncomplicated by any other serious disability.

Classification

Different terminology and classifications will continue to develop as long as attitudes towards people with learning difficulties continue to change and interest in this field develops. In the USA and Canada 'mental retardation' is the term still used, whereas the World Health Organisation and United Kingdom use 'mental handicap'. The classifications are different in other countries, e.g. 'learning disability' and 'intellectual impairment'. The following are those in use in the UK:

> Severe mental impairment – a state of arrested or incomplete development of mind, which includes severe impairment of intelligence and social functioning and is associated with abnormally aggressive or serious irresponsible conduct on the part of the person concerned and the severely mentally impaired shall be construed accordingly.

Mental impairment – a state of arrested or incomplete development of the mind not amounting to severe mental impairment
which includes significant impairment of intelligence and social
functioning and is associated with abnormally aggressive or seri-
ously irresponsible conduct on the part of the person concerned
and the mentally impaired shall be construed accordingly. (Mental
Health Acts 1983 and 1987)

Mental Health Act 1987

The Education (Handicapped Children) Act 1970 allowed access
to schools for all children who were mentally handicapped. These
schools were classified then as:

ESN – Educationally Subnormal
ESSN – Educationally Severely Subnormal

Neither of these is a valuing term, and it is to be hoped that a
more precise, valuing and appropriate classification will be used
in the future. The people themselves advocated a change of name
and decided on 'learning difficulty'. With the change of attitude
and the advent of social role valorisation (normalisation), the
expectations of people with learning difficulties have changed
radically and there is an expectation that they will learn, develop
and be accepted into society.

Chapter 3

General approach to physiotherapy

Introduction

There were physiotherapists and remedial gymnasts (as they were then called) working with people with learning difficulties for many years when it was an unpopular and unknown field to the majority of their colleagues. The profession began in 1894 with the Society of Trained Masseuses. It later became the Society of Massage and Medical Gymnastics in 1920 when it amalgamated with Medical Gymnastics. In 1942 it became the Chartered Society of Physiotherapy. Remedial Gymnasts joined the Society in 1986. Documents suggest therapists began working in institutions in the late 1960s. However, it is believed that therapists worked there even earlier. They often worked in professional isolation in large institutions which were home to 2,000 people or more, making the prioritising of 'patients' an almost impossible task.

With so much emphasis today on new attitudes to people with learning difficulties, it is difficult to visualise the problems faced by the pioneers in this field. Institutions housed children and adults from the cradle to the grave, all under the umbrella of mental handicap. With such a population there were the normal problems of childhood illness, the ageing process and its associated problems of arthritis and loss of mobility, and such diseases as multiple sclerosis and heart disease, in addition to learning difficulties; nor were they spared such epidemics as polio with its attendant potential physiotherapy needs. They also had many people with cerebral palsy and other conditions associated with mental handicap that required therapy. A formidable task.

The pioneer remedial gymnasts and physiotherapists therefore faced an enormous challenge. Before their advent there had been little or no physical therapy in institutions for those with physical problems. They had to start from scratch armed with their background training and commonsense. In those days massage and medical gymnastics was the basic area of training for therapists, followed by medical electricity and electrotherapy.

It is difficult to determine just when physiotherapists began to work in institutions since unfortunately their work was unsung and unrecorded. In the late 1950s Bobath (see p.65) was in Harperbury and Leavesden Hospitals. It is not until the late 1970s that there is a clear record of remedial gymnasts working at Fieldhead Hospital in Wakefield and physiotherapists at New-church Hospital, Warrington and Gogarburn Hospital, Edinburgh (1971). As early as 1963 a day centre was set up by parents in Stockport. Their expectations were high at that time because they wanted to prevent the deformities they saw from recurring. They used the techniques of the time, massage and movement, and they found a way of 'handling children' to help them move and to improve posture and lessen deformities. Gradually some therapists specialised in particular areas of treatment and became experts in this field.

From the 1940s specialist techniques began to be developed. Karl and Berta Bobath in England, Professor Peto in Hungary, Vojta in Germany and Glen Dolman and Carl Delacarto in the USA made major contributions to improving the quality of life of children with a physical disability.

It was the professional who had the knowledge and worked on the patient to improve his or her condition, not as today when there is a contract between therapist and patient/client for a realistic outcome to the condition. Then the expectations of the patients/clients were that the therapist would make them better as long as they went for treatment. This attitude too was fostered by the schools of physiotherapy, which trained students to try to 'cure' patients. There were other patients who would never be 'cured', but who could be helped by rehabilitation, independence training, maintenance and functional activities to improve the quality of their lives. People with learning difficulties fell into this latter category.

When physiotherapy was in its infancy institutions were re-garded as hospitals. It was therefore the practice to set up a physiotherapy department similar in many ways to a department in a general hospital. The 'patients' were taken to the department by the porters, often in the hospital transport, bus or van, because of the large area of the hospital grounds. Those people who were too deformed or too ill to be moved were seen on the wards. In addition to the problem of a large caseload there was the time taken to get from ward to ward in such large institutions, along miles of corridors or long walks in the grounds where no corridors existed.

Remedial gymnasts were innovators in this field. Their main skill was in group activities, working to establish social interaction through team work and to increase exercise tolerance by initiating sporting activities which opened new horizons for the 'patients'. Such therapists were in short supply and there were many institutions which could not employ them as they had no established posts. However, there were also institutions which would not employ them as they did not see the need for such professionals. Gradually, as the therapists' work was seen to be of benefit and as their reputation grew, more and more institutions advertised for remedial gymnasts and physiotherapists. In many institutions there was only one therapist who ran a department with physiotherapy helpers. This situation is still seen today. It is to the therapists' credit that they laid the foundations for the interest in this speciality today.

Early physiotherapy

The treatment was divided into individual and group sessions. At that time, expectations of client participation were low, especially of those with severe 'mental handicap', so treatment tended to consist of passive movements, positioning and establishing corrective seating. The priority caseload were the people with severe multiple handicaps and those with severe deformities. To appreciate the problem one has to visualise an adult with cerebral palsy and spastic quadriplegia who spends all the time lying in a supine position, either in bed or on a bean bag, and looking at the unstimulating ceiling. Due to contractures and fusion such

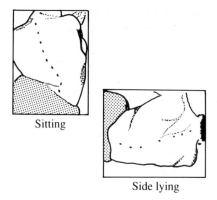

Sitting

Side lying

Figure 3.1   The importance of side lying (note correction of the spine)

a person could not flex or bend in any direction and therefore could not be seated. There would be severe flexion deformities of hips and knees and severe scoliosis (see Figure 3.1). The task of improving such positioning and giving the person a view of his or her surroundings was a Herculean one.

Today these chronic deformities are less often seen in the UK and USA because most people have had access to treatment since childhood. However, even today in some countries such as Greece and in Eastern Europe these gross deformities can still be seen because the patients (as they are still called) have little or no access to physiotherapy.

This was not the only problem facing the early therapists. They also had to face their nursing colleagues and other professionals who preferred the status quo, and who resented the extra efforts expected of them. Changing attitudes, then as now, was an uphill struggle. Finding appropriate equipment, wheelchairs, armchairs, standing frames, walking frames or even special footwear was difficult as there was not the proliferation of firms specialising in this equipment that there is today.

They had to develop skills in postural positioning, seating adaptations and types of wheelchair available. They also had to be knowledgeable in all general areas of physiotherapy as there were hospitals within institutions dealing with all aspects of client care both acute and chronic. It was important to mobilise the 'patients' who had the ability to be mobile, and much effort and skill was required by everyone involved to achieve this objective. Expectations of what the 'patients' were capable of had to be changed. If nothing was expected of people then nothing would be achieved. A vicious circle perpetuating this attitude has always worked against those with disabilities. It begins from the moment they are born when people say they will never achieve anything. This view prejudices others to have low expectations of them, which in turn deprives them of opportunites to learn. Thus, with diminished experiences they have more performance delay, and as they are not encouraged they cannot achieve their potential.

It has to be remembered that children described in the 1921 Education Act as 'mentally defective' were deemed to be ineducable and therefore incapable of benefiting from ordinary schools. The Education Act 1944 placed responsibility for the education of children suffering from 'disability of mind' in the hands of the local authorities, and special schools were established. However, severely handicapped children were excluded from school in England until 1970 when the Education (Handicapped Children) Act was passed.

Children were treated by the therapists within the institutions until the establishment of special schools when the paediatric physiotherapy service became involved. Those institutions which were established especially for children below the age of adulthood (legal age of majority varies from country to country) had schools built on site where the therapist treated the children.

Traditionally, it has always been easier to find physiotherapists with an interest in working with children than to find therapists with an interest in working with adults, especially in the field of learning difficulty. Those services which include the paediatric section still find recruitment easier.

Physiotherapists were not immune to the attitudes and expectations of their day as regards those who had learning difficulties. It was the norm to believe the 'patients' needed care like children, and that one should not expect too much in the way of learning from them. Therefore it was important to make the 'patients' comfortable, to have them sitting in the best position obtainable in order to prevent further deformities and to improve mobility where possible. Therapists also tried hard to make the sessions as enjoyable as possible, understanding and trying to compensate for the lack of continuous stimulus and interest within institutions. It is also true that people respond better to something they like doing.

Treatment of children progressed and new techniques and methods of treatment and surgery helped to prevent, limit or minimise deformity, allowing therapists to improve positioning and mobility. Here too physiotherapists had to fight to get 'mentally handicapped' children and adults seen by surgeons and to have them operated upon to improve posture or mobility. It was not considered kind to put people through this trauma when they were thought to be incapable of understanding and merely required care.

Changing attitudes

Attitudes and expectations within the service and in society as a whole have altered – some would say not far or fast enough, but change has happened. Social role valorisation (normalisation) and the movement towards community living have sparked a revolution in attitudes. Physiotherapists have embraced the new philosophy: some willingly, some reluctantly; others had always treated people with learning difficulties with the respect and dignity appropriate to their age.

Moreover, such changes are not confined to the West. Since the fall of the Berlin Wall and the opening up of Eastern Europe, former Communist countries have allowed some of their establishments to be visited. In many instances their attitudes and treatments are rooted in the past and based on the medical model of care. They require financial and multi-disciplinary therapeutic assistance to improve the quality of life of their citizens with learning difficulties. This assistance is now being given, and changes are being instigated which will benefit all.

There used to be a variance in the quality of physiotherapy practice throughout Britain. While there were many areas of good practice, there were also areas that left much room for improvement. For example, appearance is important to all of us, yet some of the orthopaedic footwear supplied to 'patients' by physiotherapists was unnecessarily noticeable and disabling in appearance.

One man, when asked why he had refused to go on a shopping trip he had previously been looking forward to, replied to the effect that his friends had teased him about his 'Mickey Mouse' shoes and he was too embarrassed to be seen in them. It was necessary for him to have surgical shoes, but with more understanding of how he wished to be seen and a little imagination more 'ordinary' shoes could have been made. It is surely understandable that teenagers, in particular, will want to look as fashionable as their peers.

While visiting a physiotherapy department, I congratulated them on an extremely well-equipped children's department and asked how many children they worked with. My embarrassment can be imagined when I was told that they only treated adults. It is difficult to believe that their 'patients' were treated age-appropriately as adults when the only equipment was for young children; nor does it say much for their expectations of the people for whom they were responsible.

In another department there was great concern for the 'mentally handicapped' patients, but the view was expressed that they could not learn and had to be looked after. A number of people were brought to the department by the porters and they all went to their usual beds; one man went to a bed in a separate room and tipped himself for his chest treatment – a learnt behaviour surely!

On the other hand, there were physiotherapy departments which developed age-appropriate activities and had high expectations of clients' abilities to learn. They introduced riding and sports activities into their already large repertoire of techniques, and worked towards more socially integrated activities in order to achieve increased exercise tolerance, function and independence.

Physiotherapy today

Client participation is nowadays expected and encouraged. All aims of treatment, work programme, management, advice or education are directed towards function and independence. These aims and objectives are discussed with the client and carer so that there are realistic expectations of the outcome. There is an understanding of the client's learning difficulties, and exercises and techniques are chosen, structured, monitored, analysed and broken down into achievable parts so that the client can achieve success and build on it.

This task analysis approach, and the expectation and belief that clients can learn, is the key to physiotherapy today. There is no place for the 'does he take sugar' syndrome.

Paediatrics

Change has occurred over the years for children who show development delay or intellectual impairment. Previously the medical advice typically offered to parents was to put the child away and forget about him or her: to leave the care of such children to those in institutions or hospitals, and to get on with their own lives. Now there is much more understanding of the grieving process that parents undergo, and help is at hand in the hospital and in the community. Community care is, however, an expensive option which must be properly funded.

In the last fifty years there has been considerable interest in the paediatric field, mainly in those with physical handicaps. Two particularly important developments have been Bobath facilitation techniques and conductive education.

Cerebral palsy is a group of conditions of great variety. In the late 1950s Karl and Berta Bobath worked long and hard to give therapists an understanding of the condition and a method of treatment to facilitate function. Bobath was the first person to establish a cerebral palsy unit within what was then known as a mental subnormality hospital.

At the 5th International Congress of Child Psychiatry in 1962 Bobath presented a paper on the experiences gained at this time (Bobath, 1963). He summarised it by saying that:

> The treatment and management of these patients seems well worth while and may help to prevent a further physical and mental deterioration of all patients while improving the physical and mental condition of some of them. Test results of intelligence expressed in terms of a numerical IQ have proved to be an unreliable guide to a patient's innate potentialities. They seem to give at best a measure of the patient's functioning level at the time of assessment. They are no guide in deciding on the desirability or otherwise of treatment. So far

the only reliable guide seems to be a trial period of observation and treatment of not less than three months.

How true this has proved to be. IQ testing has not been in favour for the above reasons for some time and observation and time are essential to allow the 'patients' to learn.

There were 'mentally defective' children's units in hospitals before schools were established. The pioneer remedial gymnasts and physiotherapists faced an enormous challenge. Before their work there had been little or no help for those with a physical problem. They had to start from scratch armed only with their background training and common sense.

Their expectations were high at that time as they wanted to prevent the deformities they saw recurring. They found a way of 'handling' children to help them move in an easier way, improve posture and lessen deformities. Gradually some therapists special-ised in particular areas of physical treatment and became experts in this field.

There was an upsurge of interest in the paediatric field in the 1940s when special techniques were developed by the Bobaths in England, Professor Peto in Hungary, Vojta in Germany, and Dol-man and Delacarto in America, who all made major contributions to improving the quality of life of the physically disabled child. These techniques permeated into schools for physically handi-capped children and gradually therapists moved into schools for children who had a learning difficulty. The new techniques became established practice. All techniques or adaptations of such techniques available to the therapist were used – Bobath facilitation, conductive education, and neurological patterning – to enable improvement to be made in the child's condition.

Every effort, allowing for the caseload and staffing levels, was made to treat children, to prevent deformities and to advise on positioning: it was always understood that the younger one started treatment, the more chance one had of preventing or limiting deformities and improving the function of the child. But when physiotherapists began to specialise in the treatment of children with learning difficulties in institutions and schools there was still much to do. Those who tried to get a child to crawl or do an exercise which would improve his or her future function or abilities would frequently encounter the attitude of 'don't be cruel, let them enjoy life'.

Parents were grateful for any help offered, and did not feel confident to challenge the professions. The professionals knew best and parental 'interference' was not encouraged. This too has changed today as parents are rightly seen as partners in the treatment, being the people who know their children best. They are the ones who will carry out the physiotherapy programme, and they are more likely to co-operate if they have participated in the planning of a realistic programme for their child. Therapists support and help parents with consultant appointments and assist in obtaining necessary and appropriate equipment and appliances.

When surgery was first performed it was difficult to get consultants interested in 'mentally handicapped' children. When they did and surgery was performed, the physiotherapists had a difficult time with the rehabilitation process. Insufficient explanation confused clients, who did not appreciate the pain or immobilisation and were not always co-operative with the rehabilitation. Unfortunately, many of the early operations on the tendo Achilles and adductors were unsuccessful due to ignorance of the problems of spasticity. Some children went 'off their feet' and others, once the adductors were cut, went straight into abduction – a frog position making sitting difficult. Spinal correction of scoliosis and kyphosis needed physiotherapist time to maintain muscle strengths, assist with positioning and monitoring the plaster cast or brace.

Adolescence

Adolescence is a difficult and painful time for most teenagers. A learning difficulty does not protect young people from the same problems of growing up as the rest of their peers, struggling to find their independence. Parents of children with learning difficulties find this time traumatic. The adult future is uncertain. Where do their offspring go after school? Will they find the same level of physiotherapy in the adult section should it be required? How can they allow the children to make decisions for themselves? The young people are wanting change, age-appropriate clothes and shoes, less noticeable wheelchairs and especially less noticeable adaptations.

Before SRV none of these problems impinged on the minds of carers or therapists as institutional living was the norm. Clothes were issued and choice was not encouraged; some establishments even had a type of uniform. The living accommodation was spacious, so the size of wheelchair was not a problem. As the residents did not leave the self-sufficient community, appearance seemed unimportant. Dressing a woman of fifty with Down's syndrome in a type of school uniform and white short socks did nothing to enhance her image or encourage adult expectations of her.

Schools too continued, and in some cases still do, this denial of the growing-up process. Nursery rhymes were often used in games or physiotherapy activity for adolescents. The 'ring, aring of roses' game in pool therapy, which began at two and was still continued at fifteen, was insensitive and unhelpful in aiding adjustment to the adult world.

Physiotherapists often work with children from the time they enter school at two or three to the time they leave at eighteen, and a close bond can be formed between the therapist, child and family. Adolescents are in many cases seen by the therapist twice a week up to the time they leave school, which leaves them unprepared for an adult world in which they are fortunate if they see a therapist once a fortnight. The parents too find it difficult to cope with this withdrawal of support and easy access to the orthodist (or maker of surgical shoes and appliances) and to equipment. Worst of all is the drastic reduction in therapy.

Today managers are encouraging closer ties between the paediatric and the adult service, and the philosophy of SRV is changing attitudes and approaches in some areas, although unfortunately much more work is necessary before this becomes the norm. The practice of having the same physiotherapist treating the same child throughout its school life is being discouraged, thus enabling the child to adjust to change and allowing him or her to experience different approaches. Treatment and approach are also becoming more age related. The therapy sessions are being reduced, but more importantly adolescents are being encouraged to take responsibility and ownership for carrying out their own programme.

Adults

It has to be remembered that therapists work not only with clients who have severe multiple problems, but also with clients who have minimal motor dysfunction, postural or balance difficulty. The physiotherapist's role in improving the client's well-being, quality of life and easier integration into society is as important in this area as it is in working with the physically disabled person. Prioritising the work in a heavy caseload is the physiotherapist's nightmare.

CASE STUDY 1

There was an account given by a man in his sixties of how he learnt to walk fifty years ago in an institution. He said that he was taken to the home when he was ten and his family could no longer look after him. On the first morning, as he staggered along the corridor, he was given a slap by the male nurse and told to walk properly. This was repeated daily until one morning he managed to walk better and the male nurse ruffled his hair, smiled at him and said, 'Well done'. This is not a method to recommend, but the man was grateful and the nurse had at least appreciated that he had the potential to walk.

With all service users, whether child or adult, the main aims of therapy are to improve function, increase independence, prevent further deformities, improve seating if required, open new horizons and introduce clients to the generic services and integrated sports facilities using whatever technique is most suited to the individual. A definite challenge!

The elderly

It would be misleading to say that all elderly people have problems that require therapy. This is patently not true as most elderly people never require treatment and live active lives until they die. It is the same situation with people who have learning difficulties. The aim with the minority that need assistance is to maintain their independence and mobility as long as possible, both for their own sake and for that of their carers, and to enable them to maintain a life with quality.

There are two areas of particular concern. First, many of the clients look younger than their years, but when the ageing process starts it accelerates rapidly, causing anxiety and confusion to the clients and carers alike. Second, Alzheimer's disease can affect people with Down's syndrome at a relatively young age – around forty – causing problems for their carers. Both these facts are of interest to people in this field, and more research is required into this ageing process.

There are other factors involved in the care of the elderly, including severely disabling conditions such as cardio-vascular accidents resulting in strokes or hip fractures and their complications, with subsequent loss of mobility and independence. These problems were not always envisaged or planned for when institutions were closed and people were moved into community houses, and this left carers unprepared and inadequately trained for such occurrences. Attention should be given to improving training for carers in this area.

The physiotherapist strives to maintain clients' independence, function and mobility as long as possible, to assist them in rehabilitation in conjunction with the generic service, to be a source of information for carers and to provide them with the skills to cope with the elderly person. It must also be remembered that the generic community physiotherapy team may be appropriate, since the elderly clients may have more in common at this stage with the elderly than with those who have learning difficulties.

General approach

The approach today is one of questioning every action, word, attitude, deed, omission, task and goal, to make sure that they match the quality standards of physiotherapy and the principles of the service. The physiotherapist should be seen as one of a multi-disciplinary group, including the client, the aim of which is to help create, support, defend and develop a valued social status for the person with learning difficulties by promoting independence function, mobility, confidence and self-value. To fulfil all the aims and objectives of physiotherapy and to assist the child or adult to achieve these aims and objectives, the most important skill required by the therapist in the specialist field of learning difficulties is the ability to teach.

John O'Brien (1987) viewed the quality of services in terms of five accomplishments:

1. Choice.
2. Community presence.
3. Competence.
4. Community participation.
5. Respect.

All these should be borne in mind when the physiotherapist is involved with a client in planning a programme of action.

Choice

Choice is a fundamental principle. People should be able to exercise control over their lives, not only in small everyday instances, but also in major decisions affecting them, with assistance when required.

Community presence

Physiotherapists should provide services in the most suitable and convenient place for the client, whether it be in the home, day centre or leisure centre; and at the most appropriate time for practice of the skill – for example, cleaning one's teeth after having a meal or before going to bed. Opportunities should be taken to work with clients, carers and the public to break down barriers to integration by increasing mobility indoors and outdoors: providing assisted and powered wheelchairs will allow those with mobility problems to go shopping, attend educational classes and integrate and participate in ordinary everyday activities, including work and leisure.

In these settings a physiotherapist is also seen as an advocate for the client, and by their actions, language, body language and behaviour in public places, physiotherapists can assist in the removal of fear and prejudice against people with learning difficulties.

Competence
People learn, develop new skills and try new experiences throughout their lives. People with learning difficulties should have the same opportunities. Physiotherapists should teach these skills in meaningful and functional ways so that the clients have the opportunity to practise and learn from their experiences.

Community participation
As people are given more opportunities to join community events in their vicinity, they develop a wider range of social contacts and relationships with other community members. Physiotherapists may initiate a contact within the community and then withdraw their support when it is felt by both the physiotherapist and the client that the client can cope on his or her own.

Respect
Respect is given when it is earned. Clients learn to have respect for themselves when they are treated with dignity and consideration and without ridicule. This should be evident in the physiotherapist's manner from the moment contact is made with the client, in the way the physiotherapist addresses the client, conducts the discussion about the referred needs and provides an explanation of what intervention would be suitable. The client should feel valued and be seen by onlookers to be valued.

Clients have a right to live in the community as independently as possible, interacting and co-operating with their peers, colleagues and other community members. When they are seen to have the opportunity to participate in community activities and have valued roles within the community, they will lose the negative stereotyped image of 'mental handicap'.

CASE STUDY 2

Arthur L

Mr L was a young man in his early thirties with learning difficulties, a poor memory and a physical problem with hemiplegia who could only walk short distances when assessed. He lived at the time in an institution which was planning for his move into the community. This became of concern when it was realised that he tired easily when walking to the nearby shops. It had been assumed that Mr L's exercise tolerance would be greater as he was often seen walking around the large grounds of the institution. This is a common assumption which overlooks the fact that in an institution people stop to see friends, watch what is being done around the grounds or simply sit down and have a rest when they are tired. They might only walk about 75 metres without stopping.

Mr L was referred to the physiotherapy department available at the time in the institution. He was assessed and time was taken to get to know him and to find his strengths (which were many) and his needs. Walking to the shop was not sufficient exercise for Mr L; nor was it particularly interesting or enjoyable, which made him reluctant to go.

The therapist involved wanted to find a meaningful way to engage Mr L in activities which increased his exercise tolerance, afforded him enjoyment and if possible provided him with a hobby. The therapist was determined to give Mr L choice, to help him to participate in the community by using public facilities when suitable, and to teach him the skills required to engage fully and appropriately in such activities.

The aims and objectives were discussed fully with Mr L, appreciating that his experiences were limited. An explanation of the programme was given, and short- and long-term goals were discussed and set. The goals set were as follows:

Programme	Targets
Exercises in gym progressing to Circuit training	4 weeks
One-mile hike/walk around local woods (short-term aim)	1 month
Five-mile hike/walk on specific nature trail (mid-term aim)	12 months

Outward bound activity week   18 months
(long-term aim)

The programme was considered totally unrealistic by some carers and many colleagues who believed that the expectations were too high and that such activities involved an unacceptable risk. Teaching is not just showing a person how to learn and perform a skill; it also needs to be a skill that will enhance that person's image, be valued by others and elicit admiration and respect. It is unfortunate that people with learning difficulties have to prove this point.

To give Mr L the opportunity to accomplish what he set out to do, he joined an activity group run by the therapist which was tailored to the individual's ability. He gradually progressed to circuit training, thereby increasing his exercise tolerance. He was reluctant to use his left arm, he had perceptual problems affecting his balance and he also suffered an increase in muscle tone when under stress.

All the exercises were stepped back to a point where he could accomplish them, and this success encouraged him to become motivated and competitive. An important rule of teaching in this area is not to allow failure. Unfortunately, failure is a feeling too often experienced by clients, and one which saps their confidence.

Walking began a month later with members of Mr L's group. Not only did his exercise tolerance increase and his balance improve, but he also used both hands in pushing branches out of his way and when climbing over trees. The five-mile hike was achieved within the time span allotted and Mr L's carers were as pleased as he was. It changed their view of him and opened up new opportunities and horizons. Similarly, outward bound week was a great success and Mr L was supported when he applied to join a rambling club.

Not all teaching has results which raise awareness so spectacularly. Some results seem small, but to the individual involved they are monumental.

The five accomplishments of the service were all achieved in this situation:

1. Throughout the teaching Mr L was given realistic opportunities to make his own decisions.
2. Activities were carried out in suitable and convenient settings.
3. Mr L was taught the required skills so that he could participate fully in these activities.
4. The activities took place within the community and there were opportunities for making new friends.

> 5.   As these activities were seen by society as valuable, respect was given to Mr L for his achievements, in addition to the respect he earned by his determination and efforts to accomplish each task.

Other considerations

Cultural and religious views influence how people are seen and treated by their society. It is necessary for therapists to appreciate, understand and respect this even if such views do not coincide with their own. Without this knowledge much harm can be done unintentionally with parents and carers to the detriment of the child or adult with learning difficulties. As the multicultural and multiracial society develops, therapists will encounter this situation more often, and to be able to achieve the aims and objectives of their programmes for the child or adult concerned, they will have to develop a precognition of the situation so that everyone involved will work for the same result.

Many changes have occurred in the Health Service, especially in England following the White Paper 'Working for patients' and the opportunities it has given for some hospitals to apply for and achieve trust status. The formation of health trusts and provider and purchasing units is changing the pattern of service provision.

Services for people with learning difficulties may be delivered from an acute trust or community trust, or may remain district managed. It could be more difficult to protect the specialist services in this new environment. It is therefore all the more essential that physiotherapists prove that the service they are providing for the client is value for money. Physiotherapists must measure and record progress so that an outcome measure can be costed.

References

Bobath, K. (1963) 'The prevention of mental retardation in patients with cerebral palsy', *Acta Paedopsychiatrica*, vol. 3, no. 4, pp. 141–54.

HMSO (1989) 'Working for patients. The Health Service: caring for the 1990s', White Paper, London: HMSO, Cm555.

O'Brien, John (1981) *Principles of Normalisation: A foundation for effective services*, London: Campaign for People with Mental Handicap. Adapted for CMH by A. Tyne.

Chapter 4

Specific physiotherapy treatment

Introduction

The aim of the physiotherapist in the service for learning difficulties is to improve physical performance where there is functional
deficit, using various means to motivate, stimulate and facilitate
so the client will achieve and fulfil his or her potential.

This can be done by direct intervention using specific techniques: provision and maintenance of seating, wheelchairs, special
footwear, splints or mobility aids. It could include hydrotherapy,
hipotherapy or rebound therapy. Or indirect intervention can be
used, i.e. teaching and advising others on a number of subjects.

The role of the physiotherapist is as follows:

1. To provide a functional and clinical assessment when required
   and appropriate.
2. To evaluate the assessment and provide a programme plan of
   work based on the client's strengths and needs.
3. To implement this programme.
4. To monitor its progress and evaluate the whole intervention, identifying possible development work required for the
   future.

To do this with children or adults who have a learning difficulty
where does one begin? In exactly the same place that one would
start with anyone who needed to be seen by a physiotherapist –
with an assessment. From this assessment it is possible to develop
an individual programme plan for the client and to monitor the
success of treatment in achieving the desired outcome.

The importance of assessment

Assessment may take half an hour if it involves giving advice on how to access the generic service; or it could take many sessions, months in fact, getting to know the person, winning their confidence and establishing a rapport with them before satisfactory assessment is achieved. Although it is important to move away from the medical model of care to the social model of care, there is no substitute for an assessment. The difference comes in what the programme is, and how it is followed through.

There are some questions to be considered before beginning any assessment. This enables the physiotherapist to obtain the correct information about the referred problem and to be able to formulate a precise programme plan.

1. Why is the assessment necessary?
2. What purpose does it serve; how will intervention make a change to the person's life?
3. Who is the assessment for?
4. What changes will occur in the growing and developing child, especially with spasticity?
5. Are there the resources to fulfil the aims and objectives of the finished assessment?

In the case of people with learning difficulties it is said that there are extra considerations to be observed in accordance with the social role valorisation philosophy. I would dispute this as I believe the following considerations should be extended to all.

6. Has the agreement or consent of the child's parents or the adult been obtained?
7. Have the relationships around the client been taken into consideration?
8. Is the approach holistic?
9. Are the person's rights being infringed in any way?
10. Is the approach suitable in speech and attitude to the age of the person to be assessed? (We can be very patronising to the elderly.)
11. Is the approach positive?
12. Is there privacy?

13. Will the assessment and the method of assessment improve the person's status?
14. Has confidentiality been assured?
15. Has the risk-taking aspect of the approach and the activity to be pursued been taken into consideration?

Many types of assessment forms and charts have been devised by therapists to suit the specialised techniques they have developed. Other assessment forms suit different conditions, mobility difficulties and environments, and different methods of working. Unfortunately, no one assessment form is suitable for all, so there has to be some compromise to find the most universal one, especially when patient audit and quality assurance monitoring are part of the health care package.

Most assessment forms are problem orientated, which makes them most suitable for the acute service. This is not how one wants people with learning difficulties to be seen. Such a negative approach, seeing the client as a problem, is not helpful; nor does it lead to high expectations from the child or adult. Problem-orientated medical record (POMR) has combined the best of most assessments and is the most universally used assessment form in the acute sector.

Most assessment forms when examined closely are really checklists which help formulate a logical approach to investigating a child's or adult's difficulties or needs. An assessment form which uses a person's strengths and needs leads to what was originally called an individual programme plan (IPP), now known as a programme or plan for individual needs (PIN).

A 'strength' is something a person does well – or an asset which he or she possesses. It includes activities the child or adult might enjoy, and their existing skills. It is easier to motivate people through an activity they enjoy. A 'need' is something the child or adult would benefit from learning to do, a functional activity, better balance or learning to use a powered wheelchair, for example.

The objective is to alter the negative approach to those people with learning difficulties, to view them as people who have some skills which can be built on. Not only should attitude and approach be positive, but consideration should also be given to the way in which notes are written up. Take the following description of a young woman:

> A 26-year-old woman, spastic quadriplegia with severe mental retardation, epileptic, incontinent, requires specially adapted wheelchair, dependent for all her needs on carers.

This paints a negative and unhelpful picture of the person and can colour others' perception of her. The following description might have a different effect:

> An alert young woman of twenty-six, with spastic quadriplegia and learning difficulties, sitting in a wheelchair and showing an interest in her surroundings. She has episodes of epilepsy and incontinence.

Individual programme plan

The individual programme plan (IPP) approach started in the USA in the mid-1970s, and then spread and developed in many countries. Nimrod in South Wales developed IPPs for their clients from 1980, and IPP is still the basis for most systems in England. To achieve an overall policy district-wide, many health authorities set up working parties to establish agreed ways of working and to plan staff training programmes. It has to be remembered that the medical model was used when hospitals for 'mentally handicapped' people were the norm, and case conferences were the only arena for discussing the problems and future plans of the 'patients'. The client was rarely, if ever, involved at that stage.

Programme for Individual Needs

PINs are based on personal growth and are particularly suited to chronic long-term problems. Clients are involved with the carers and the multi-disciplinary professionals in planning their individual programmes. The intention of individual planning is to improve service-based provision for people with learning difficulties by identifying their strengths and needs, planning to co-ordinate the services required and tailoring these services to the consumer.

While using the same basic principles, the precise format of PIN differs between health authorities. Table 4.1 is part of a PIN from

Table 4.1   A programme for individual needs (PIN)

Areas to be considered	Strengths	Needs
Health		
(a) Are there any significant issues regarding [X]'s general health?		
(b) What assessment/advice is required, e.g. regular hearing/eye tests, medical/surgical/orthopaedic appointments?		
(c) What special equipment/adaptations (hearing aids, glasses or dentures) are required?		
(d) What support does [X] need with any of these?		
Choices		
Does [X] express any preferences concerning health issues, e.g. weight, wearing glasses/hearing aids, smoking, visiting doctor. Are these choices informed choices?		

one health authority. It sets out questions which, when answered, will build up a picture of the client's strengths and needs.

Once the physiotherapist has formulated plans from the assessment, the PIN is completed with the participation of the client. An example of part of an individual's PIN is shown in Table 4.2. The mobility section has been chosen as this is one of the relevant areas to the physiotherapist. The concern at this time was the client's 'painful hip', which was being investigated. When the PIN has been completed, a meeting will be arranged with the client and all those staff and multi-disciplinary professionals involved with providing a service for him or her. From that meeting aims and objectives will be set and the physiotherapist will set goals and timescales (see Table 4.3). These physiotherapy goals and time scales will be monitored by managers at appropriate intervals when doing clinical audits. In this way goal-setting and time scale skills will be improved.

Table 4.2 Completing the PIN (Segune)

Mobility	
Strengths	Needs
1. Segune has a matrix seating system placed in a Barrett 10 wheelchair	Sequne needs his matrix seating to be reviewed in the light of his posture changing because of the lateral movement of his hip joint.
2. Segune enjoys movement. He is able to roll and change his position whilst lying down. Can prop himself up on his right arm into a half sitting position.	Staff need to be aware of Segune's enjoyment of movement so that he is given the opportunity to use his floor mat.
3. Given adequate support around his pelvis, Segune can sit for short periods of time on a bench.	Segune needs total support for lifting. All staff must be aware of the need for Segune to be lifted correctly to save stress and discomfort on his hip joint.
4. Segune attends hydrotherapy sessions and works very hard. He is given the opportunity to gain awareness of his body – the cause and effect of movements – and to improve relaxation.	Staff need to ask for suggestions and advice on physical activities, positioning and movements, so they can assist Segune during these sessions.
5. Segune goes to a centre once a week where there is an area suited for him to try more physical activities.	Segune needs to have opportunities to change his position regularly.

Components of assessment

In terms of suggestions for physiotherapy treatment, the following assessment headings are relevant:

1. Reasons for referral.
2. Observation.
3. Communication.

50 Specific physiotherapy treatment

Table 4.3 Segune's physiotherapy

Goal	Time scale
1. Organise appointment for matrix seating to be changed. Forms filled in and sent.	2 days
2(a) Communicate with keyworker and staff on type of movement Segune enjoys.	Ongoing
2(b) Plan programme for mat activities – and teach to carers.	2 weeks
2(c) Plan programme with client and keyworkers for centre activities and teach to client and carers.	4 weeks
3(a) In-service training for new staff on lifting and positioning.	Within 6 weeks
3(b) Update lifting and positioning.	Within 2 weeks
3(c) Monitor lifting and positioning.	Ongoing

4. Sensory assessment.
5. Social situation.
6. Past experience.
7. Physical assessment.
8. Functional assessment.
9. Adaptations and special equipment.
10. Medical considerations.
11. Areas of concern.

Reasons for referral

The assessment depends on the reason for referral: for example, the client is unable to sit unsupported, is unable to crawl, has unsteady balance, cannot transfer (i.e. move from one chair to another, bed to chair, etc.) or cannot cope with stairs. It will then focus on the referred need, non-developmental progress or loss of function. Perhaps the carer is finding it difficult to lift or transfer the child and requires help.

The assessment of referred needs may have different priorities according to those involved:

1.   The client.
2.   The referrer.
3.   The physiotherapist.
4.   Other agencies.

For example, Mr Keogh is a gentleman in his forties with Down's syndrome. He has been referred by the carer at the home which he shares with two other men because he cannot get in and out cf the bath without help.

1.   The client does not see this as a priority as he always receives help when he needs to have a bath.
2.   The carer's priority is the problem of lifting Mr Keogh in and out of the bath and the back problems this causes him and the other staff.
3.   The physiotherapist's priorities are to see what physical problems, if any, prevent the client getting in and out of the bath unaided and then to find a way for the client to overcome them. Another priority is to see that the staff know the correct transfer-assisting or lifting procedures.
4.   The other agencies:
     (a) The occupational therapist is awaiting the outcome of assessment before supplying bath rails, a special bath or recommending a shower.
     (b) The housing association is awaiting the decision to see what alterations might be necessary to the bathroom, and the financial implications of this.

These priorities would be discussed with all concerned, and after the assessment a decision would be made about the aims and objectives of the planned programme.

Observation

Much can be learnt from observation. It is an area that physiotherapists need to cultivate with people with learning difficulties, and it is as important to the assessment as touch.

Is the client male or female?
Is the client young or old?
Is the client alert, lethargic, apprehensive, etc?

Is the client mobile?

If not, is the client wheelchair dependent? What type of wheelchair is used? Is it suitable for the client's needs? Does it detract from the client's image? Is it safe?

Does the client have eye contact?

Is the client moving his or her hands, and if so, are the hands used functionally?

Is the client listening to what is being said? Can he or she hear what is being asked of them?

Is the client interested in what is being said?

What is the client's respiration like? (Note this especially with children who have cerebral palsy as it has implications for exercise and eating ability.)

How do they communicate – with eye contact, verbally or with sounds?

Observe the relationship between the client and the carer. Is it positive or negative? Listen to how they communicate. Does the carer have positive expectations of the client; does the carer expect the client to learn? How the client is moved, held or lifted all contribute to a picture of the client–carer relationship. Considerable information can also be gathered without disturbing the client in any way while being introduced and getting to know him or her.

When writing observations down give a brief description of the child or adult using positive image projection. For example, take the following two descriptions:

1. A middle-aged man sitting in a chair and looking through a book.
2. A man with Down's syndrome looking at a colouring book.

Example (1) would be a more positive description as the man is more important than his syndrome; the syndrome may be required later and can then be introduced. The colouring book is not age appropriate, but this may not have been his choice and may say more about the carer's attitude than the client's choice.

To attain all the information required for a full assessment the physiotherapist must be conscious of the need to formulate many questions. Some of these can be answered by observation; others will need to be asked of the client where possible, or the carer where necessary.

Communication

Verbal and non-verbal communication
What type of communication does the client use? If *verbal* communication is used, what type is it? Is it with speech or sound? What strength is it, and of what duration? What concepts does the client understand?

If *non-verbal* communication is used, is it eye pointing? Is facial expression used, or gesture (hand pointing, shoulder shrugging, etc.)? What language is used – Makaton signing or Rebus illustrations?

During the assessment the therapist needs to observe the following:

Vision and looking
   Can the client maintain eye contact?
   Can the client track a moving object? (This skill is necessary to be able to use eye pointing as a method of communication.)

Control of hands and arms
   Can the client grasp and hold objects?
   Can the client use both hands equally well?
   Can he or she point?
   If the client can use the hands in any of the above ways, there is a possibility that he or she could communicate by using gesture.

Hearing and listening
   Can the client hear? Does he or she look towards the person who is speaking?
   Can the client turn his or her head to look in the direction of sound? If not, could the client be deaf?

If the therapist is concerned that the client might be deaf, a hearing test may be requested. The test can be difficult to conduct, however, as many clients do not co-operate with the audiologist. The Brain-Stem Evoked Response, although time consuming, has been of great benefit to clients with learning difficulties. Sedative or anaesthetics are not essential, but can be administered in cases where it is to the client's benefit.

Control of speech musculature
    Can the client suck? (Observe this when eating and drinking.)
    Does the tongue protrude?

Breathing
Children with cerebral palsy may have shallow and irregular breathing, often interrupted by intermittent spasms which cause them to breathe through their mouth. This will interfere with the production of sound and eating and drinking.

Vocalisation
The client may make many different kinds of sound in an effort to communicate, and it is important to give time to listening and learning those sounds that have meaning.

Expression of emotion
Expression of emotion is another means of communication. It can denote pain or distress, joy, happiness or anger. Is the client's expression of emotion used in an appropriate manner and at an appropriate time? It may be necessary to question what the client has been taught, since children are sometimes taught to smile for 'Yes'. How do you say, 'Yes, I have pain' by smiling?

It is important to ask the person being assessed if they use pictures or symbols to communicate. If this is the case, the communication book or card should be used.

The next step is to discuss the child or adult with his or her speech therapist to gain a better understanding of the situation. The method of communication that the client is learning can then be used and reinforced when working with the client. This will also help prevent confusion for the client.

It is essential to prevent a situation where practitioners in the different disciplines do not know the objectives of their colleagues. In one school a child had been taught by the speech therapist to look to the right for yes and to the left for no. The physiotherapist wanted him to look up for yes and down for no. His teacher had another method! It is unfair and unproductive to expect someone with a learning difficulty to learn three ways to say yes and no. Communication applies to all disciplines.

Sensory assessment

Vision

Can the client see? Does he or she wear glasses?

If the client has a vision impairment, what type is it?

One vision impairment is only being able to see out of the corner of one eye when holding the head at a certain angle. This has great significance in assessing posture and the position of the head. In one case a physiotherapist was insisting on good head position without understanding that this correction would prevent the client from using the small amount of vision he had.

There are some simple but helpful ideas that can assist the visually impaired client. For example, a different colour marking on the edges of stairs and doors in the school, the home or in departments would make life easier for all. There is also a correct way to hold and assist the client with mobility. There are many societies and associations for the blind and visually impaired which promote better understanding of this disability, and which are of assistance in training the therapist to have more knowledge of clients' needs.

Hearing

A high percentage of people with learning difficulties have a hearing loss which in many cases has gone undetected for many years, thereby causing increased learning problems or even misdiagnosis.

Can the client hear?

Is the client profoundly deaf, or is the hearing impaired?

What sounds can the client hear (frequency, volume, duration)?

Does the client wear a hearing aid? If so, a reminder when it is not in place can be helpful to a client and the carer, especially if the client requires assistance placing it in the ear.

Physiotherapists have no training in this area and speech therapists who do have these skills can be consulted. The comments in the previous section on communication are also relevant here.

Sensation

> Can the client taste and smell?
> What is the client's pain tolerance?
> Is there any sensory skin loss?
> Are there any areas of hypersensitivity?
> Is the client tactile-defensive?

The latter condition is occasionally found in people who have lived in institutions for many years, especially children. Due to lack of staff or time, they often received little touching or cuddling compared to the amount that most children receive, and they developed a reluctance to be touched or to touch objects or people.

This is an area which would benefit from more time and research.

Social situation

Where does the client live? Does he or she live with parents, with foster parents, in a children's home or institution, in shared housing with friends, in a social service hostel or independently?

What is the housing situation like? A home visit may be necessary to understand the home conditions and the level of support that the client receives, so that all programme plans will be realistic as to space, equipment and assistance available. Adaptations or alterations may be necessary to improve the client's mobility or function. Close liaison with the occupational therapist is necessary in this area.

What relationships are important to the client?

Does the client have an advocate?

What are the client's likes and dislikes? It is much easier to motivate people to do something they like.

What hobbies does the client enjoy? This is another area through which function can be improved.

Past experience

A knowledge of the client's history, which has helped to shape his or her present experiences, is helpful to the therapist when assessing the client's abilities and planning a future programme:

1. From nursery, ordinary or special school. (Each would give a different perspective on life to the young adult.)
2. From college, day centre, workplace or retirement home.

Physical assessment

Depending on the client's needs, the following information may be required.

1. Range of movement, patterns of movement, spasticity and muscle tone.
2. Type of deformity: for example, scoliosis, kyphosis, decreased range and the subsequent limitation of movement.
3. Body awareness, spatial awareness and perception difficulties.

Functional assessment

The functional assessment should include an appraisal of the following:

1. Daily living skills.
2. Mobility.
3. Ability to walk.
4. Ability to get in and out of the bath.
5. Ability to climb stairs.
6. Ability to transfer from one place to another, e.g. bed, toilet, car.

Adaptations and special equipment

Physiotherapists are involved in providing necessary, useful, safe and functional equipment throughout the age spectrum, often in conjunction with their colleagues in occupational therapy. Always check your legal responsibilities in the provision of safe and appropriate equipment.

Environmental situation

Is there room in the house, and can the family cope with the extra standing frame, special seat, trolley, etc. for a client?

CASE STUDY 3

On a home visit there was considerable difficulty getting through hallways with all the equipment that had been provided for the client. The mother was embarrassed and upset. The house was small, and with two other active children not only could she not use all the equipment, but she was prevented from using the essential piece because the rest took up so much space. The parent already felt guilty, and now she was made to feel inadequate and incompetent as well.

Does the equipment provided still perform its function? Without monitoring there are occasions when the equipment has outlived its usefulness.

Do chairs, wheelchairs, etc. conform to legal requirements? For example, foam and material covering must meet fire regulations and also be correctly labelled. Safety is a particularly important concern with second-hand equipment and appropriate labels are essential

Wheelchairs

Wheelchair assessments can be carried out by physiotherapists or occupational therapists depending on custom and area. Assessment requires knowledge, sensitivity and understanding of the person's needs, as well as patience, lateral thinking, adaptability and sheer determination to afford the person with a comfortable, functional and presentable wheelchair at the end of the day.

The objectives of all therapists are as follows:

1. To identify people who have mobility problems and complex needs which necessitate aids such as wheelchairs, special seating and adaptations, and to assist them in obtaining appropriate and necessary equipment.

2. To provide assessment and advice so that a wheelchair is supplied which will attain the mobility required.
3. To teach the correct, safe use of such equipment to clients and carers.

It is the supplier's responsibility to check that the equipment is safe, sound and functional when it is delivered. The supplier or manufacturer should also inform the wheelchair user of the name and address of the repairer and the necessary maintenance involved.

Many books cover in considerable detail assessments for wheelchairs and the types of wheelchair available. There are some basic rules when assessing a person for a chair.

1. *Reason for referral.* Is the loss of mobility temporary (e.g. fractured leg) or permanent (e.g. multiple sclerosis)?
2. *Considerations.* These should include user's wishes (colour, type, style, etc.); lifestyle (independent or dependent); activities (hobbies, sports, etc.); carer's wishes (e.g. elderly infirm parent); and accommodation (accessibility, space).
3. *Diagnosis.* On most request forms for a wheelchair the person's diagnosis is required. In the service for learning difficulties, however, it is not always possible to give a definite diagnosis and therefore the type of disability is more commonly used.
4. *Physical assessment.* This includes weight, height, physical deformities, visual impairment, sensation loss and pain. For example, sensation loss is a cause for concern because of pressure areas which may require a special cushion within the wheelchair itself.
5. *Functional assessment.* This includes the strengths and needs of the wheelchair user: the user's ability to transfer, his or her physical ability to use a manual/powered wheelchair, and his or her posture/balance (e.g. a seat belt or postural support may be required). It also includes the client's level of independence and need for assistance. It is important to maintain independence and confidence for as long as possible.
6. *Medical considerations.* Is the condition of the user stable

or deteriorating (e.g. a person with a learning difficulty and multiple sclerosis)?

7. *Environmental and social factors.* These include the type of accommodation (e.g. ground floor or high rise); accessibility (ramps, lift, door widths, etc.); location (terrain); and transport.

8. *Type and size of wheelchair.* There are a variety of wheelchairs on the market. Some are automatically supplied by the local health authorities, but here there is a limited choice. Manufacturers are at last designing lightweight, colourful and custom-made chairs which can be purchased by the user privately.

9. *Measurement of user* (see Figure 4.1)
   (a) Length of lower leg, from the bottom of the heel or shoe heel to the back of the knee (popliteal fold).
   (b) Distance from the bottom of the buttocks to the olecranon when the elbow is comfortably flexed (90° angle).
   (c) Distance from the bottom of the buttocks to the armpit; subtract 10 cm (4 in.) to give the distance to the scapulae.
   (d) Widest distance across the hips (or thighs if larger) and shoulders.
   (e) Distance from the rear of the buttocks to the back of the knee.

10. *Measurement of chair* (see Figure 4.2)
    (a) Distance between the top of the seat or cushion and the footplate or floor. NB: measure the height for transferors.
    (b) Armrest height from the seat to the top of the armrest.
    (c) Height of the backrest.
    (d) Seat width; allow 5 cm (2 in.) for additional clothing.
    (e) Seat depth; subtract 7 cm (3 in.) to avoid pressure at the back of the knee – if the full measurement is used the canvas of the seat will dig into the back of the knee causing pressure sores, etc.

11. *Other considerations.* You should aim for symmetry and distribution of load bearing through both ischial tuberosities and the whole of the thighs and buttocks. Pelvic tilt should be avoided where possible (i.e. the pelvis should be neutral), as should asymmetry (e.g. windswept hips, scoliosis). Provide

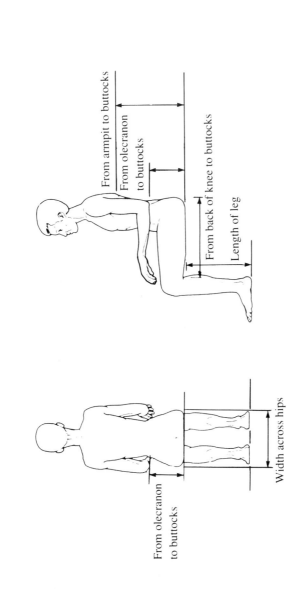

Figure 4.1 Measurements of the wheelchair user

Height of armrest
from seat to
comfortable armrest
position.

Seat depth minus
7cm (3 in.)

Width of seat
(allow 5cm (2 in.) for
clothing)

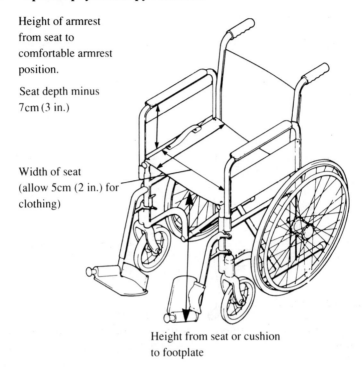

Height from seat or cushion
to footplate

Figure 4.2   Chair measurements

appropriate support to stabilize the pelvis and lower limbs in
all the postures being considered. Then, once the lower part of
the body has been stabilized, determine the postural support
required at the trunk level without diminishing functional
ability.

With people who have severe deformities it may not be possible
to achieve much of the above. However, it is important to give
the user as comfortable a seating position as possible. It may
be that the client will require a body support inset, such as a
Matrix Mould or Derby Mould, to fit into the wheelchair. If this
is necessary, it is vital to choose a chair which will accommodate
such an adaptation safely.

Medical considerations

What medical conditions are present which can affect the client's programme?

What drugs has the client been prescribed?

What knowledge does the therapist require to work with someone who has epilepsy or hepatitis B?

It should be noted that neither of the latter should prevent the client taking part in most activities, including sport. Nor should they be discriminated against because of these factors. When clients first went to use a swimming pool all was well until it was realised that some clients had 'fits' and there was an unnecessary scare about hepatitis B. It took some time and explanation to relieve this fear, and the clients now continue to use the pool, enjoy their hobby and learn to swim without further problems.

Areas of concern

From assessment findings the following problems may be discovered:

1. A wheelchair could be unsuitable or unsafe.
2. Scoliosis could be developing.
3. There may be hearing problems to follow up.
4. The client's behaviour may challenge the physiotherapist, who may need to find out more information and learn how best to work with the client.
5. The relevant information from other disciplines may not have been received.
6. If there is a lack of physiotherapy staff to carry out the required programme, how and where is this service deficiency recorded?

Plan and programme

With the assessment completed the next stage is to set out the aims of the programme. These are then discussed with the client and the objectives are set. If necessary, these are divided into short- and long-term plans. Time scales are also set. It must be remembered that intervention may consist only of the provision of a walking stick or advice, or it may mean long-term intervention over a number of years.

Task analysis

Whatever the programme, each objective must be broken down into the smallest components so that the client can understand and achieve each stage, and build upon his or her success to reach the final goal. The approach must be consistent, and the language used should be comprehensible to the client and simple without being patronising.

Monitoring

Evaluation of the client's progress is essential so that each stage can be assessed and the next stage added or adjusted and taught to the client and carer. If a lifting programme has been taught, this must be updated and monitored to prevent bad practice occurring through familiarity.

The decision to discontinue the episode of care is not always an easy one, especially with increasing caseloads and pressure from parents and carers. This is why the assessment is essential and skill is required in setting objectives and time scales.

Quality assurance measures (see pp. 71–5) also need to be monitored to maintain a high-quality service.

Techniques and skills

Traditional attitudes and methods of working do not always apply when working in the area of learning difficulties, which adopts a social model of care rather than a medical model. Physiotherapists need to make changes not only in their practices but also in their attitudes towards the client group.

At the beginning of a time of change there is often a feeling of insecurity and lack of direction, and anxiety that core skills will be lost. In fact, all the skills that physiotherapists command can be called into use at some time in this specialist area; a generalist background is very useful in this field. The skill lies in choosing the appropriate technique for each individual in order to obtain the optimum results. It is also important to be able to teach a client who may appear to be unmotivated and unresponsive.

In the field of learning difficulties it is essential to work in a place which is appropriate and will have some significance for the person involved. There is little point, for example, in climbing stairs in a physiotherapy department when these go nowhere and bear no reality to the stairs in the person's environment. This can be confusing for someone who is learning the 'normal' pattern of living in the community. It is only acceptable if the person is a patient in a hospital.

In the paediatric section the aims, objectives and techniques are somewhat different, although function and independence must be the eventual objective. It is detrimental only to see the child and not to see the future adult within. The very young child, especially one who is multiply handicapped, will need assistance to improve balance, head control and mobility, and to prevent deformities – the developmental approach is appropriate at this stage. As the child becomes a teenager and then an adult, the therapist needs to alter the approach by using age-appropriate language and activities, as well as social integration and social interaction. Discos may be enjoyable for most teenagers, but most elderly people prefer a less noisy environment.

The particular choice from the many techniques which the therapist has to treat the client, and to advise, manage or teach the parent or carer, depends on the ability, interest and training of the physiotherapist. This book does not aim to give detailed descriptions of every technique since it would not do justice to them; it seeks only to make the reader aware of the methods available in the hope of stimulating interest and research.

Some treatments have limited aims, such as relaxing spastic muscle or increasing postural stability at a joint; other treatments have a global approach which takes on the role of a philosophy of treatment. The age of the child also dictates the type of treatment as co-operation is essential in some areas.

The Bobath technique

The late Dr Karl Bobath, a neuropsychiatrist, and Berta Bobath, a physiotherapist, began their life's work with brain-damaged children in 1943. From the Bobath Centre in England they worked with children who had cerebral palsy from all over the world, and they lectured and ran courses in many countries. Their techniques changed and evolved over many years with experience. The emphasis has changed, but the basic concept has not.

It is understood that in cerebral palsy neurological lesions lead to interference with the normal maturing processes of the brain, causing abnormal reflex activity which leads to abnormal posture and movement patterns.

Some of the features of the Bobath technique are as follows:

1. Reflex inhibitory patterns are used to inhibit abnormal tone associated with abnormal movement patterns and abnormal posture.
2. Learning movement through the sensation of moving. The child with cerebral palsy knows the sensation of abnormal movements and cannot use any others.
3. Facilitation techniques are used to mature postural reflexes for the initiation of movement. There are key points of control (where the physiotherapist holds the child to control her movements).
4. Working is a team effort, with parents and carers involved in the total management and life of the child, to gain a holistic approach to treatment, advice or management. In this way the planned programme is carried over into everyday routine, preventing a fragmenting of the client's life into separate compartments.

In neuro-developmental disorders there are no straightforward approaches. David Scrutton (1984) suggested some criteria by which these diverse treatments might be classified:

1. Mechanical: based on muscle power, joint range, line of gravity base, mass and postural stability. It naturally leads to treatments which influence these factors and is probably the most easily understood approach.
2. Neurological: based on different aspects of neurology: peripheral, utilising exteroception and proprioception to facilitate or inhibit muscle action; and central, which by a variety

of means and to different degrees sets out to influence the disorder or the effect of the disorder by changing, if not the structure, at least the function of the damaged central nervous system.

3. Educational: in which intervention becomes more akin to 'education' than 'treatment'.

Conductive education

Conductive education, introduced by Andreas Peto, falls into this last category. It originated in the Institute for the Motor Disabled in Budapest, the motto of which is 'Not because but in order to'. It is goal orientated and has positive expectations of the child which are shared by the parent and conductors. The conductor is specially trained as a generalist and many physiotherapists have had such training. Conductive education is a programme of learning which has a repetitive, consistent approach that is helpful to those with learning difficulties.

In an institution recently a young woman was referred to a physiotherapist because 'she had gone off her feet'. During the assessment it was realised that the school she had attended had used a modified conductive education approach. She was then asked to stand using a form of words used by the conductors: 'I will stand up. One, two', etc. She immediately remembered the words, and using the sequence and rhythm formula she soon became mobile.

Lifting

Most physiotherapists would rather this was not part of their role today; it is time consuming, difficult and fraught with legal complications, codes of practice and legal standards. Much discussion has taken place as to who should be responsible for the teaching of lifting: should each profession be responsible for lifting within its own speciality? This debate will continue, and it is up to the individual and the service to try to clarify the situation.

Clients with physical disabilities who need to be transferred or lifted have the right to expect a comfortable, safe, painless and injury-free move. Physiotherapists have skills which would enable these criteria to be fulfilled, and when necessary they should teach them. In the field of learning difficulties one has to be aware that a client's behaviour may be unpredictable, which could add an extra dimension to lifting and the use of hoists.

It is not enough to teach lifting alone: how to touch, hold and move a client must also be part of the main lifting package. So too must be the safety of the carer.

The package should include the following:

1. District or service policies.
2. Legal guidelines pertaining to lifting.
3. The principles of lifting.
4. Anatomy tailored for the group to be taught. Obviously the details will differ according to whether the group consists of multidisciplinary professionals, volunteers, parents or whoever.
5. Types of lifting appropriate for the client group.
6. Techniques of lifting.
7. Types of wheelchair; how to fold and afford easier lifting.
8. Types of adapted seating, moulds, etc.
9. A practical session.
10. The paperwork involved: course content, signatures, etc.
11. The future monitoring of the lifting taught.

Demonstration
A demonstration of the techniques of transfer and lifting should be given, and attention drawn to touching, holding and particularly client involvement. Every interaction the physiotherapist has with people with learning difficulties should further their knowledge or ability in some way, whatever the ability level happens to be. The client should participate in the lift, if only by initiating, leaning forward in the wheelchair or moving the head. This must always be expected before assistance is given. Clients will gradually improve on any movement, be it with a quicker response time or a more definite movement.

Practice
Once the techniques have been demonstrated, these should then be practised and experienced. At a recent teaching session for

carers in the hydrotherapy pool, the number of comments from the carers when they were lifting and moving each other, and the discomfort experienced when they were being moved, increased their awareness of the importance of correct technique.

If the carer's lifting technique is not suitable or safe, this must be recorded. If the physical condition of the carer gives cause for concern, this must also be noted, the carer informed and the relevant manager told that in the therapist's opinion that carer is unsuitable for a lifting task. In the case of parents, the therapist would need to advocate on their behalf for assistance from community services.

Written records of practice sessions should be taken and kept. Each country will have its own criteria for records, and physiotherapists must be familiar with the legal requirements. The following data are suggested:

1. The place where lifting occurred.
2. The date of lifting and the actual time it took place.
3. The length of time the session lasted.
4. Attendance. Names, places of work and managers of those attending should be kept, together with the names and designations of physiotherapists taking the lecture.
5. Course content. The learning objectives should be clearly stated, and the information shared and the skills demonstrated should be listed. Anything the trainees are taught not to do should also be recorded, e.g. 'Never lift on your own.'
6. Practical sessions. It is important to note the competence or otherwise of individual course members in the practical skills. Inform managers of any gross inability to perform safely a practical skill at end of a session. This should be recorded.
7. Records. These should be kept for seven years. The time scale should be checked as this may vary from one district physiotherapy service to another.

Lifting should be seen where possible in the environment in which the carers work. This enables the physiotherapist to see the ergonomic situation and to adapt the lifting to the individual client.

The legal limits on weights to be lifted vary between different countries, and different policies on the lifting and handling of loads have to be taken into consideration and followed. Care must be taken to explain the difference between transfers and lifting techniques: lifting always requires two people, whereas a transfer does not because clients take some weight and some responsibility for themselves.

CASE STUDY 4

Mr Agege

Mr Agege was an elderly man with a learning difficulty. While temporarily in hospital it was assumed that, because he was non-verbally communicating and had a learning difficulty, his comprehension would be low. He was therefore not asked to help himself and was lifted in and out of bed. Mr. Agege enjoyed the extra attention and did nothing to remedy the situation. The team therapist liaised with her colleague in the hospital and the situation was rectified – much to Mr Agege's dismay as he now had to do more for himself.

The hospital physiotherapist, when discussing Mr Agege's discharge with the carers, said that he had to be lifted. This was reported back to the team and caused consternation. They could not provide an extra carer to assist with lifting; nor could Mr Agege remain in the warden-controlled flat where he was living, since he would need a higher level of support than before and this would not be provided. He would therefore have to move.

The team therapist contacted her colleague immediately as she was sure that there was some misunderstanding. This was resolved when the therapist was contacted and explained how the confusion had occurred. She had assumed they would understand that she meant Mr Agege could transfer! This misunderstanding over the distinction between transfer and lifting nearly cost Mr. Agege his home and friendly neighbours.

Children are easier to move, but one must remember the weight lifting specified. (The EEC Manual Handling of Loads Directive gives directions on health and safety requirements when lifting, particularly with a view to preventing back injuries.) Lifting and moving children may also be part of their treatment programme, especially when they have cerebral palsy. Correct lifting and holding can inhibit muscle spasm and facilitate movement. For example, holding a child in a flexed position during carrying inhibits extensor spasm and facilitates a better head position.

If hoists are used, make sure that these have been properly demonstrated by the manufacturer and that all those who manipulate them are properly trained.

The ergonomic situation must be carefully assessed when lifting in the home, school, swimming pool or ski-slope environment, so that a safe, comfortable lift or transfer can be obtained.

Quality assurance

One of the dictionary definitions of 'quality' is excellence; 'assurance' can be defined as a promise or pledge. Thus, quality assurance involves promising excellent service standards.

The concept originated in manufacturing industry to improve the standard product in order to reach a level of excellence in the most effective and economic way. It is a procedure by which standards are specified for work done, and these are monitored to check that they are maintained.

Quality assurance has been the main preoccupation of those in health care in recent years. The Health Service is in the business of producing and promoting good health. Physiotherapy manufactures treatment, intervention and management advice for the customer (client or patient) at a specified standard in order to produce a desired outcome, be it mobility, positioning or independence.

A 'quality circle' is a group of people within an organisation who meet together on a regular basis to identify, analyse and solve problems relating to quality, productivity or other aspects of day-to-day working, using problem-solving techniques. Quality circles originated in the USA and were then transported to Japan. The first Japanese quality assurance circles were formally recorded in 1962, creating improvements in the quality of Japanese products and thereby increasing the demand for the country's exports.

Quality circles have now been set up in the Health Service, sometimes producing surprising results. For example, a quality circle was set up in a ward for the elderly. One of the results of this was a return to 'proper' crockery: cups, saucers, milk jugs and teapot. The ward had previously been using a tea trolley, dispensing tea and coffee into plastic cups. The elderly people who had complained of this were delighted with their new-look teatime. They looked forward to their tea and drank more, and teatime became a social occasion. Fluid intake increased, kidney infections dropped, fewer drugs were required and the time spent in dealing with infections fell. It therefore proved to be both cost effective and a huge moral booster to the elderly people involved.

Most quality measures will fall within five main categories

1. Legal requirements: guarantees of adherence to codes of practice, service policies and statements of intent.
2. Provision of systems to ensure quality: audit, supervision and consumer opinion.
3. Setting standards of both general and local concern.
4. Setting specific clinical outcome measures.
5. General assumptions: reasonable expectations of standards of work provided by the physiotherapist and his or her practice.

A statement of intent or philosophy for the service should be drawn up. For example, the physiotherapy service believes that people with learning difficulties have the same basic human rights as the rest of the population. Therefore they should receive a service of high professional quality tailored to their individual requirements. It should be delivered in a way that adheres to the five accomplishments for enhancing and advancing the clients' physical needs and well-being.

The criteria by which quality is judged should include the following:

1. How to access the service.
2. What range of physiotherapy is provided.
3. What clients and carers think about the service they receive.
4. What policies are available: complaints, risk taking, sexual and equal opportunities for service users, etc.

The audit

Each service, department, school or community physiotherapy service should have a standard which states what information is essential to provide the therapist and the service with an insight into the client, the environment in which he or she lives and the relevant medical information. The assessment plan of intervention, time scales and the needs of the client should be clearly stated.

A set of criteria for an audit needs to be established. This should state what information must be recorded to provide that service with the tools to make a reasoned judgement on the client's abilities, strengths and needs. Some notes are required by law, and they should be clearly recorded so that another therapist can extract the essential information required when taking over the care of the child or adult.

Each service sets its own criteria for audit. These typically involve some of the following:

1. Name and address of client.
2. Name and address of referrer.
3. Date of assessment.
4. Diagnosis. (This is important in the paediatric section, but less so in the adult section, where in many cases it is not known).
5. Assessment.
6. Plan.
7. Programme.
8. Time scale.
9. Name of therapist assisting.
10. Signature of physiotherapist.

Data collection and storage

Well-organised data improve our understanding of problems and help us to take decisions wisely. In many areas of physiotherapy attempts are still being made to work out the appropriate information to store on computers. This will supply the service with useful information to assist physiotherapists and their managers with their work. It should also assist in supplying this information quickly. However, accurate information depends on the quality of the raw data. There are also policies of confidentiality concerned with putting notes on computer disks, etc.

Standards for physiotherapy attitudes

These are difficult and subjective to qualify. It has been frequently shown that there is a wide variation between what we do and what we think we do. John Badenock (1986) highlighted the dangers of even the most experienced clinicians assuming that they knew all about their own behaviour and the impression they gave others.

Physiotherapists should adopt the following attitudes:

1. Use a friendly approach, making the client feel respected and at ease.
2. Treat each person in a manner appropriate to his or her age, and as a worthwhile individual.
3. Listen to what the client says or tries to say; use signs or Rebus to help facilitate communication and respond appropriately.
4. Do not make the client feel hurried.
5. Grant privacy and dignity to the client in speech, touch and dressing.
6. Recognise the client's right to make decisions for him or herself, even if this is to refuse physiotherapy.
7. Remember that a difficult or awkward client may be fearful, upset or worried; try to help resolve these problems.
8. Be sensitive to cultural backgrounds and aware of the resulting differences in attitudes to learning difficulties, so as to eliminate misunderstanding from the beginning.
9. Be aware of the rights and fears of parents and carers, be sensitive to their attitudes and tactful in suggesting change.
10. Understand some parents' inability to let go of their children at any age and their need to foster dependence in their children. Sensitivity, tact and patience will be required in this situation.
11. Encourage realistic client participation in all aspects of the physiotherapy programme. Do not always assume 'I know best'.
12. Take care in both the spoken and written word not to use devaluing labels or to make the diagnosis more important than the person.
13. Be aware of confidentiality in discussing and note taking, and do not leave notes in inappropriate places or disks in word processors.

Clinical specialities have produced their own quality indicators. According to Barnes *et al.* (1989) the physiotherapy service should accomplish the following for the client:

1. Physical integration.
2. Social integration.
3. Individuality.
4. Autonomy and protection of rights.
5. Positive image and role status.
6. Capabilities and competence.
7. Continuity.

References

Badenock, J. (1986) 'Communication in medical practice', *Journal of the Royal Society of Medicine.*

Barnes, J., Dennis, C., Barrell, A. and Jenkins, J. (1989) *Standards for Good Practice in Physiotherapy Services for People with a Mental Handicap*, London: Association of Chartered Physiotherapists in Mental Handicap.

HMSO (1990) EEC Manual Handling of Loads Directive, adopted 29 May 1990, for implementation by 31 December 1992.

Scrutton, D. (ed.) (1984) *Management of the Motor Disorders of Children with Cerebral Palsy*, Oxford: Blackwell.

Chapter 5

Treatment, advice and management

Introduction

Treatment, advice and management are each easy to define. But whatever intervention a physiotherapist chooses to use with a client, it is perceived by others as 'treatment'. We are still haunted by the medical model.

Treatment is the hands-on work that physiotherapists do with clients in a one-to-one situation using whatever skills are necessary to attain a satisfactory outcome. Treatment tends to be primarily within the paediatric section. It diminishes towards adulthood and is sporadic within the adult sector.

Advice is given to a wide range of people – clients, carers, voluntary agencies and the public – on such varying subjects as how best to look after physical disabilities, choose a wheelchair or access public facilities.

In 1949 Sir Charles Renold stated that 'management is a process of getting things done through the agency of a community'. An important element in physiotherapist working practice is to get things such as the planned programmes done through people – the carers. This requires good management skills and tactful persuasion.

There is a great deal of discussion on the appropriate methods of intervention in physiotherapy these days, but physiotherapists have always believed in the correct intervention for a specific individual. They have seen the client as an individual with individual needs, fears and abilities which have to be improved, resolved, comforted and changed using whatever means of individual attention are necessary. At different times in the client's life there will be a need for treatment, advice or management, or all three at the same time.

Treatment of the client's condition, management of the client and carers, and advice to carers or other agencies on a large range of subjects are all part of the physiotherapist's role. Physiotherapists are aware that resources are scarce and that the demand for their services will exceed their resources. Prioritising of caseload is therefore essential in this area.

With the pressure of workload it is important not to attempt to take on more clients than can be accommodated. The reason for intervening in a client's life is to provide an effective physiotherapy outcome, be it increased mobility, better seating or improved comfort. To be overstretched provides neither the client nor the therapist with any degree of satisfaction.

Learning difficulty is not a disease but a condition which can be associated with physical disabilities: with chest complaints, decreased mobility, diminished perception, contractures and deformities. These may be acute or chronic conditions.

Acute conditions should be seen in the generic services in the same way as the rest of the population. Little acute work is provided in the adult section of the physiotherapy service, except when there is a hospital situated within the institution where the clients receive all their medical attention. In the paediatric service it may be desirable to keep the child out of hospital in order to prevent separation from the parent and increased anxiety for the child.

The main role of the physiotherapist in this situation is to be advocate for and on behalf of the client in accessing the generic services. Even when the client is admitted to hospital, the physiotherapist should be available to give advice on management and the abilities of the client should this be necessary.

CASE STUDY 5

Pat S

Ms S was a lady in her fifties who had cerebral palsy and developed an acute chest infection while living in an institution. The physiotherapist there had been monitoring her condition and informed the GP of his concern. The response was to do nothing; the GP claimed that the physiotherapist was available for her treatment and therefore there was no need for concern.

It was pointed out that there was no weekend cover and that if Ms S had been living in the community she would probably have been admitted to hospital. Eventually Ms S was admitted to the local hospital and liaison took place between the two physiotherapy services.

The physiotherapy managers of both the hospital and the service for people with learning difficulties arranged, if necessary, to call into the hospital a physiotherapist from the learning difficulty service.

Ms S had been in hospital for two days when her physiotherapist was called in for advice because of her deformities, perceived inability to communicate and difficulty with drinking. Ms S was also unhappy as no one talked to her, took the time to allow her to initiate any movement or helped her to obtain a position in which she could drink. These difficulties were overcome by explanation of some of the problems that people with learning difficulties experience, particularly with time delay.

The correct sitting position for Ms S, which inhibited the extension spasm, was demonstrated; this allowed her to drink more easily. The way in which the therapist communicated with Ms S also showed the ward staff that Ms S could understand and was interested in her surroundings. However, the staff found this non-verbal communication difficult to cope with, and Ms S had a lonely stay in hospital.

Children with respiratory conditions are often seen in their homes by the physiotherapist as this is less disruptive and disturbing for them. Many children with disabilities spend an inordinate length of time in hospitals and attending hospital clinics, which can have the effect of institutionalising them. Hospitalisation for children is both frightening and emotionally traumatic, disrupting their normal life and giving them a distorted view of the world.

When chest conditions occur the children are treated at home whenever possible. They receive breathing exercises and postural drainage. These exercises are then explained and taught to the parent, who continues the exercises and management for as long as necessary. The physiotherapist monitors the situation at intervals.

The physiotherapist's role within this service is to provide advice to clients on their long-term disability and to help them to work towards their full potential in terms of health, increased mobility and function. As movement specialists, we are not simply concerned with how a limb moves or how a person walks but also have an obvious interest in how movement and mobility is used in everyday life.

Intervention techniques

Many specialist techniques and models have evolved over the years to cater for the complex problems arising from central or peripheral nervous system dysfunction. Some physiotherapists specialise in one particular technique; others use a more electic approach, employing whatever system will benefit the client.

In an attempt to analyse the approaches used by physiotherapists in neurological management, Gonella et al. (1982) reduced the basic principles of all techniques to four, while conceding differences in conceptual emphasis and procedure:

1. Use of sensory input to facilitate or inhibit the central nervous system.
2. Application of neuro-developmental concepts.
3. Application of skilful manual techniques.
4. Use of concepts from the psychology of learning, such as conditioning, reinforcement and response generalisation.

Here we see again the application of mechanical, neurological and educational techniques.

The following techniques are used within the service for people with learning difficulties.

Bobath

The concept of 'neuro-developmental treatment' is based on two factors:

1. The interference in the normal maturation of the brain by the lesion, leading to the retardation or arrest of motor development.
2. The presence of abnormal patterns of posture and movement, due to a release of abnormal postural reflex activity.

The Bobath method aims to give the child the experience of more normal posture and movement, by the treatment of abnormal postural reflex activity through inhibition, in order to facilitate movement. It is realistic, influenced by the disability of the client and should be used as an integral part of the client's management programme.

Kabat

Herman Kabat, working with Margaret Knott and Dorothy Voss, developed a system of movement facility and methods for hypertonus inhibition. Methods were based on mass diagonal patterns, sensory stimulus to facilitate movement, and resistance to movement in order to increase the action of muscles. The concept of movement patterns used in proprioceptive neuromuscular facilitation is used in physiotherapy and was described by Knott and Voss in 1968. Special techniques are rhythmic stabilisation, repeated contractions and the hold–relax method. This technique has its uses within the service.

Doman and Delacato

Glenn Doman and Carl Delacato worked with Temple Fay at the Institute for the Achievement of Human Potential, where they pioneered a technique to give the individual visual and tactile stimulation with increased frequency, intensity and duration. The aim was to allow the child 'unlimited opportunity to function in full recognition of the orderly way the brain grows'. The technique follows developmental sequences, and it includes patterning, which requires a continuous team of helpers. The technique's heavy dependence on volunteers, and the pressure it puts on the parents and the rest of the family, make it a difficult and stressful option. However, some parents believe it to be essential for their child's development and make a heavy commitment in time and money to carry on with the method. Should the regime break down and the child return to school, it is important to understand the parents' needs and to deal sensitively with them.

Conductive education

Andreas Peto developed this method of combining therapy and education together as an inseparable homogenous unit:

> Positive expectations on the part of the parents and conductors are important but also the child's body image, his self concept and the child's perception of his environment. It is future or goal orientated not focussing on the past or the etiology of the problem. A dysfunction is not the property of the child but the product of the interaction between himself or the way he is and his environment or the way he is perceived. The primary aims of conductive education is to stimulate developmental process and is performed by conductors who are specially trained.

Some physiotherapists have been trained in the conductive technique.

Physiotherapists need to have considerable experience of many modalities when working with learning difficulties, so that each referral of a client will receive the specific technique suitable for the condition presented. While it would be impossible to practise all these techniques, physiotherapists should at least be aware of them, and the alternative therapies such as reflexology and acupuncture practised by some physiotherapists. It is important to remain open-minded and to refer to colleagues who have the skills needed for the client.

Physiotherapists must only use techniques they are trained in and which they are competent to employ, and no two problems are alike. For example, a child with cerebral palsy resulting in spastic quadriplegia requires:

1. Movement to prevent contractures.
2. Posturing to prevent deformities.
3. Seating to allow the child to be aware of his or her surroundings.
4. Movement to assist towards whatever function is possible.

Bobath facilitation would inhibit extensive spasm and achieve a position from which the child could work towards head control or hand movement; or another method might be chosen which would suit a particular individual and therapist.

Another child could be referred with ataxia, requiring work on balance, function and activities. In this case conductive education might be the method chosen by one therapist, while another therapist might choose another methodology. It is also true that many techniques and parts of techniques are chosen to provide the client with an eclectic approach to his or her need.

So-called 'clumsy' children who have minimal dysfunction are often under stress because they are always being told not to knock things down, or bump into doors, or trip upstairs. Advice should be given to carers on:

1. Perceptual problems.
2. Body image difficulties.
3. Inability in some cases to cross mid-line.

Such advice, as well as recalling the simple fact that the child is not just being careless, can help to ease the stress of the situation.

With this understanding the carers can take the pressure off the child and the physiotherapist can begin with exercises aimed at improving spatial awareness and body image. These can be incorporated into the child's physical education routine and the child's teachers can continue with the management of the programme. At intervals the physiotherapist will monitor, evaluate and update the programme.

Management

Paediatrics

As children are in school most of the day, advice on how to achieve the best results for them using exercise programmes and positioning should be part of the school routine. It is important, therefore, that teachers, carers and bus attendants are aware of why children are seated in certain positions, and why children are held or moved in a particular way. These skills have to be explained, demonstrated and taught to the carers so that when they are confident and competent the management of the child can be handed over to them. It must be understood that this will be monitored at intervals and that carers can always call the physiotherapist in for advice when they need it. In this way co-operation can be obtained and the routines continued throughout the day to reinforce the therapy input.

Adolescence

At this stage the planned decrease of treatment should have progressed to a point where the sudden withdrawal of therapy does not cause distress to client or carer, and the young person is guided towards being responsible for his or her own management and function. Monitoring may be provided at weekly intervals, extending to monthly or biannual intervals when advisable, thus preparing the child and parents for the adult service. However, some severely disabled children may require some physiotherapy at intervals throughout their lives.

By this time spinal correction may have been performed, and when the young person returns to school this may require monitoring or management of the situation. The physiotherapist may be required to visit the consultant with the child if there is a problem.

Adults

In the adult sector treatment is sporadic, but management has a higher profile. Trained carers maintain the agreed programme, which is monitored and updated periodically by physiotherapists. Liaison with the social services is invaluable at this stage as they may be providing services into the client's home and their staff should know the necessary programmes.

The elderly

The elderly require little treatment. Occasional rehabilitation may be necessary to maintain mobility. It is sometimes deemed to be less traumatic for clients to be treated in their own homes rather than go back and forward to an outpatients department, which could be confusing and traumatic.

Elderly people have problems with osteoporosis which can result in fractures and cause difficulty within their home. If the Community Service cannot help or if the client is too challenging, it may be more appropriate to have the physiotherapist from learning difficulties monitor the rehabilitation, and teach the carers the necessary skills to enable them to manage the situation.

Alzheimer's disease sufferers have very short memories and forget where they are, causing extra problems for the carers. There are cases of people with Down's syndrome developing Alzheimer's disease in their forties. Elderly demented clients challenge the system and the carers. The carers need support from the physiotherapist and help to improve their skills in assisting elderly clients. The transfer or lifting techniques might require updating, and assistance may be required in helping the client to keep mobile.

Clients who have even mild cerebral palsy find ageing unhelpful to the condition and may 'go off their feet'. This will require a period of rehabilitation either to regain function or to assist the client to adjust to wheelchair dependency. The carers will need help and new skills to accept and cope with this new situation.

Carers are often unprepared for cerebral vascular accidents when they occur, and will again need assistance during this anxious time. This may take the form of advocacy on behalf of the client when he or she goes into hospital, so that the client's learning difficulties and non-verbal communication (if this is unaffected) are understood. The changes, both physical and emotional, should be explained to client and carer, and whatever physiotherapy intervention is warranted in this case should be given when the client returns home from hospital.

One of the most time-consuming areas of physiotherapy advice is in the provision of shoes to assist clients who have foot deformities. It is essential for clients to have comfortable, presentable and age-appropriate footwear. This needs energy, imagination and patience, as well as some lateral thinking. In one case boxing boots have fulfilled a need for a client who has severely deformed feet and habitual routine behaviour of removing any footwear. These also look more in keeping with the style of the day!

Clients of all ages with challenging behaviour also need treatment for their various conditions. The reasons for their aggressive, unsociable or unacceptable behaviour need to be understood. The causes may be considered as falling under three main headings:

1. Personal circumstances.
2. Environmental circumstances.
3. Home circumstances.

The personal circumstances could include frustration due to lack of communication, being imperfectly understood if they have a speech impediment, or being unable to make their actions understood. They may be unable to articulate the simple pain of toothache or backache, physical discomfort, hunger or thirst, or even when their clothes are too tight and they are unable to adjust them. Perhaps they find the weather too hot, too cold or too windy, and perhaps they are incorrectly dressed for it. Again, the clients' inability to communicate these feelings may make them frustrated.

Environmental circumstances may include overcrowding in a room or on transport, or too noisy, confusing or distracting an environment. Insufficient space can oppress and irritate the client, causing anger and discomfort.

In the home, rows can elicit understandable fear and anxiety in the client; illness of parents or staff can cause worry; and separation, being moved from people they care about or their home environment, often without explanation, can add to a client's anger and inability to understand a situation. Not being told when someone they care about dies, and the grieving process at their loss not being understood by others, is another cause of anxiety in clients.

Understanding the reasons for such behaviour means that the client can then be treated appropriately. If an instance of aggressive or difficult behaviour occurs, the physiotherapist should remain calm, caring and responsible. The client's attention might be diverted and the situation gently defused. The physiotherapist should try to establish calm by use of body language, unthreatening eye contact and voice level, tone and pitch.

Fear and anger are unhelpful in this situation. It is important to concentrate on the person and not the attitude. Before one works with a client, it is helpful to know if there are any trigger situations which can cause increased agitation. Get to know the client and do not push them beyond the point where they have had enough. Activities can always be gradually increased later.

CASE STUDY 6

Justin O

Mr O was a large and active young man with non-verbal communication who could be gentle but had occasional aggressive outbursts. Unfortunately, his reputation had gone before him, making his physiotherapist apprehensive when she was asked to see him. The clinical psychologist's advice was sought, and she suggested calm and consistent behaviour. She pointed out that he did not like his feet being touched and that this needed to be understood.

Mr O was referred because it had been noticed that he had some muscle wasting of his hands and feet. His carers' advice was taken on the best time and place to see Mr O, and a meeting was arranged. It would take a period of weeks to get to know, observe and finally assess Mr O, but after the initial assessment it was obvious that the muscle wasting did need investigating. An appointment was made with the neurologist.

The assessment continued over the weeks while waiting for the neurologist's appointment. The calm, consistent approach worked well, and the behavioural modification programme set by the clinical psychologist was followed. Mr O co-operated more as he got to know and like his physiotherapist.

The physiotherapist went to the hospital with Mr O and his carer for the appointment with the neurologist. Mr O was not subjected to an overcrowded, noisy waiting room, which would have confused and frightened him in the new surroundings.

When during the examination he became agitated, the situation was quickly defused by everybody behaving in the same calming way. Mr O relaxed and the examination continued.

Mr O needed the condition monitored over a six-month period, and this was followed through without difficulty.

It is rare for a physiotherapist to have to cope with violence. However, the following important points should be considered, if the need arises.

1. Bear in mind organisational factors, such as district guidelines, legal advice and managers' responsibility.
2. Know the warning signs and understand the difference it can make being on a client's home territory and being on the physiotherapist's territory. Choose the best location for both participants.
3. Plan for the worst scenario so that if a difficult situation arises there is a pre-planned way to respond. Always know where the nearest exit is. It may be better to withdraw in some cases for a while as long as the client will be safe and will find the quiet calming.
4. When a therapist is involved with such a client their line manager should always be informed and know when and where the session will be.

If the physiotherapist is in any doubt about being able to work with clients who challenge the service it is important not to do so, although extra training might be sought. This is a specialist area and, although rewarding and very important, only therapists with the skills and interest can competently obtain the desired results.

Passive or active treatment?

Passive treatment is perhaps a misnomer. It was used to describe the manipulation of a movement in a client who took no part in that action him or herself. This does not increase function or independence, although it was and is used to gain full range of movement and prevent contractures. Only in massage is the client expected to be passive and relax and not 'do' anything, especially when the therapist is trying to reduce tension.

In every treatment or activity a person with learning difficulties must have some active participation, no matter how small. The amount will depend on the ability and the condition of the client, but it is essential to foster and enable choice, power and responsibility within the client. If a client is wheelchair dependent with no visible means of activity, this is the first area to work on. Can the client move his/her eyes? Lift his/her head? Move his/her hand or finger? Once this is established, treatment starts to make the client conscious of having some control over how he or she is moved, through whatever means of communication the client has.

Eye movements, if consistent, can be used for 'no'. Depending on the linguistic understanding of the client, the speech therapist might advise the use of eye pointing for one response only. Once this can be used consistently, a 'yes' can perhaps also be added.

It would be too much to expect a client to initiate a head movement from the supine position. Begin where it will be most easily achievable: almost sitting, so that the client can lift his or her head and try to lean forward, thus helping to initiate movement. From being able to bring the head slightly forward, work to bring the shoulders forward. The physiotherapist may assist the client to place his or her hands in the lap, again in a position which will assist the shoulder movement. Each step is taught carefully to the client using language concepts that the client understands and leaving time for the client to accomplish the task.

This method is explained to the carer and the reasons for the process given. This co-operation is essential so that the treatment can be used in the appropriate place at the appropriate time: when getting out of bed into the wheelchair, getting into the bath, etc. Each time there is a lifting or close adjustment to be made, the client should initiate the movement by use of the head.

The step-by-step approach continues until the client can lean forward when lifting is necessary, and therefore has some small autonomy in the situation. As the client's movement increases, the assistance given can be decreased. The starting position can also be changed as the client masters each stage, until the client can initiate the movement from the supine position, if that is realistic for them.

The main aim of treatment, advice or management is to attain a satisfactory outcome, by achieving goals set out in the programme plan for the client. If this is not achieved, the physiotherapist must re-evaluate the programme:

Where or why was it not achieved?
Were the time scales unrealistic?

Was the intervention chosen the correct one for that client?
Was the method of teaching unsuited to the learning curve of
the individual?

Never be afraid to evaluate the programme and to re-assess the
goals set and achieved. Do not undermine your abilities by setting
a goal so low that you are always seen to achieve. When the outcome is not as satisfactory as planned, check the process, find out
what prevented the client and therapist achieving, and learn from
the result. The outcome should be discussed with the client and
manager if necessary, the goals reset and the necessary corrections
made. The goals will be achieved next time, and confidence and
skills will grow with experience.

References

Gonella, C., Kalish, R. and Hale, G. (1982) 'A commentary on electromyo-
graphic feedback in physical therapy', *Physiotherapy*, vol. 68, no. 2.
Knott, M. and Voss, D. E. (1968) *Proprioceptive Neuromuscular Facilitation*, London: Harper & Row.

Chapter 6

Teaching

Introduction

Teaching is a skill unfortunately not taught at the moment in physiotherapy schools, but a skill more and more necessary for physiotherapists today, when clients are party to the contracts of therapy required. In addition, parents and carers need to be taught an understanding of the programmes provided in order to ensure their participation and continuous input into the programme for the child or adult involved.

Teaching may be defined as the stimulation of learning; and it is an active process conducted through doing, reacting and undergoing. In this way the learner participates in his or her own education.

The first requisite of teaching is knowledge, but although essential, knowledge alone is not enough. Teaching involves the ability to impart this knowledge to others in a comprehensible, easily assimilated way. Some people have a natural aptitude for teaching; others have to work hard to cultivate it.

The scope of teaching

The opportunities for teaching are many, and they apply at all stages in a physiotherapist's career from the treatment of the first patient to lecturing to a large audience of multi-disciplinary professionals on subjects as diverse as specialist technique and business management.

In the service for people with learning difficulties, teaching occurs in all of the one-to-one situations that take place with the client to facilitate ongoing learning. However, physiotherapists are also involved in the following aspects of teaching:

1. Training the carers.
2. In-service training
3. Student education.
4. Public relations.

To be effective in the service of learning difficulties the therapist must have an interest in initiating, guiding and motivating the child or adult to learn, and the therapist must be enthusiastic and encouraging as the client strives to acquire new abilities or to improve old ones. Explanations have to be given at a level that can be understood and in a language that is comprehensible, using signing if necessary. Tasks should also be achievable: success and deserved praise are the stimulus to endeavour and learning. This approach to teaching is important when working with people who learn slowly and find learning difficult.

The therapist has to believe that learning will occur, and should use lateral thinking (i.e. if the first method does not work, try another), problem solving and any other consistent method which will increase the learning curve of the individual. Someone once said, 'It is not they that cannot learn, but we who cannot teach.' This is a heavy responsibility, but one that is worth carrying. Watching someone learn and enjoy learning is the reason why working in this speciality continues to hold excitement for those involved.

One method that has been successful in this area is *systematic instruction*. This was conceived by Marc Gold in Los Angeles in the late 1960s, and by the early 1970s he was lecturing on this technique in the United States and Canada. The method has undergone a process of change since then and it has enabled clients to learn complex tasks by building up competences brick by brick. It has proved to be a powerful tool in training people with learning difficulties to do marketable tasks for employment and is now used in many countries.

Systematic instruction is worked on a one-to-one basis and each task is analysed and broken down into component parts. The client begins the task at the appropriate stage for him or her, and as the client's competences develop assistance is gradually reduced. In this way the client acquires a number of competences in a systematic way.

Whatever method is used, it must take into account the nature of learning and the different levels of maturity of the learners. The aims and objectives of teaching are the same throughout the age spectrum, be it for clients, parents, relatives, carers, students or colleagues. The outcomes of learning are the absorption of facts, new skills and fresh attitudes, and the appreciation of others' abilities.

Physiotherapy is a scarce and expensive resource and one that must be used effectively. To do so therapists must employ their skills to assess needs to make the necessary decisions on which modalities to use, to plan programmes, to treat with hand-on skill when necessary, and to pass on certain skills to carers. These carers will, it is hoped, have the time, the interest and, when taught, the ability to continue with the programme, thus releasing therapists to do the work for which only they are trained. This is a most cost-effective way of working, involving a good skill mix and developing the skills of others.

Carers

Carers are a variety of people who care and provide for people with learning difficulties, helping them to take their place in society and to live as full a life as possible. They range from long-term carers like parents, spouses and partners, and some staff in those institutions still in existence, to short-term carers like those employed to assist a child through nursery and school life and those employed to support adults in their home, in the community and in the workplace, or helping to facilitate integration in all social settings and activities.

Parents and families

Physiotherapists in the service for people with learning difficult- ies have many opportunities for working in partnership with parents, and this requires different skills for each age range and each area of work. From the moment the child is born with a multiple handicap, parental involvement is essential and care and sensitivity are required in assisting the parents to hold, move and cope with their child. Physiotherapists must remember that their competence in this area can make an already anxious and diffident parent feel even more inadequate when they find this handling and movement quite difficult to begin with.

Realistic support is vital in the early stages to lay a firm foundation for future progress. An understanding of the emotional trauma felt by the parents and families of children diagnosed as having a learning difficulty, and those with the multiple 'handicap' of physical disability, should help to formulate the approach used in this area of teaching. The rest of the family can also be shown how to carry on the programme devised. Success can be measured when the parents and family are confident and competent with the child and the programme.

Parental involvement may continue throughout the client's life, and teaching may also continue at various stages as the need arises, to assist the client to be as independent as possible. Some parents find it hard to believe that people with learning difficulties attain their majority at the same age as other young adults and that they have rights, one of which is to accept or refuse physiotherapy intervention.

School teachers

Nursery school is the next step. Here teachers and care attendants need to understand the physical problems presented by children with learning difficulties, and how to allow the child to participate as fully as possible in all the activities available. When the time arrives for the child to attend school – state, private or special school – the physiotherapist's report, stating the child's abilities, needs, programme and relevant medical information, should be sent to the next physiotherapy service involved. This report will be part of the baseline from which the programme at this school will evolve.

Here the therapist will use whatever techniques and treatments are appropriate. Handing on these skills to the key workers, teachers and carers is essential so that programmes are continued and incorporated into the child's daily school routine. Children grow and find new strengths, they have new needs that require new planning and programme-setting, staff changes occur – all of these necessitate an ongoing programme of teaching and monitoring throughout the school life of the young person.

Leaving school is frequently a traumatic experience not only for the client, but also for the parents and even for the physiotherapist who has become attached and concerned with the young person for whom they have been responsible as part of the school team. Reports go to the next school or day centre or the private physiotherapist to ensure continuity of care, be it supervision, physical intervention or management. If possible this changeover should be planned for at least a year before the client leaves school so that the school therapist can consult with the therapist in the adult field and exchange information and ideas. This situation can call for sensitive handling, since physiotherapists too can feel threatened by a change of approach and perhaps by new attitudes and expectations in the adult service. In order to achieve a smooth transition there needs to be tolerance, open-mindedness and co-operation between the services. This problem does not arise, of course, in services which are all-embracing of children and adults, although here it may be difficult to adjust to an adult approach when of necessity most of the physiotherapist's time is spent in the paediatric section.

The community

Teaching continues in the adult service, to provide those involved with the skills to help adults keep the abilities they have acquired, to gain more if possible, but always to participate in all the activities available and attain a good quality of life. Most adults have hobbies and interests in which they become involved and which give them a worthwhile social life; so too should people with learning difficulties. Physiotherapists can be involved in the initial stage of these activities where realistic support is vital. This could involve teaching some skills themselves, or advising others on physical disabilities and expectations both for and of clients. Advice is sought from and given to sports centres, swimming clubs and outward bound centres, concerning the ability of clients to use the facilities to the full and adaptations which would assist physically disabled clients to participate.

Caring for the elderly is not an easy task, and with an emphasis on care in the community more and more people will be struggling with elderly relatives. It is not unknown for parents in their late eighties to be caring for their handicapped son or daughter in their fifties; it has also been the case that a son or daughter with learning difficulties has looked after an elderly parent. In this area, physiotherapists become involved in teaching carers in the home, in social service agencies and in voluntary agencies the skills required to help people remain mobile and as independent as possible throughout their lives. In cases where an elderly client's needs are solely to do with age, advice or treatment should come from the community therapists in the generic services, since the elderly person with learning difficulties has more in common with other elderly people than with other people who have learning difficulties.

Teaching such a variety of people requires time, commitment and ability to impart the required information at the correct level, at the right time, and in a way that is interesting, stimulating and hopefully memorable.

Client teaching

Skill exchange must be taught in many different venues. If we are concerned with teaching the client however, this must occur in the appropriate place and at the appropriate time for it to have meaning and value to the individual and so that he or she will be receptive. If we are concerned with teaching the carers, this must take place in the home, school, day centre, residence or place of work as the therapist is responding to the referred need. For example, if getting in and out of the bath is a problem, then the client needs to be taught that skill in a bathroom, so that the teaching is meaningful and functional. People with learning difficulties would find a hypothetical situation confusing and meaningless – in fact a deterrent to learning.

Physiotherapists have a wealth of information on anatomy, physiology, medical and surgical conditions of treatment, techniques and interventions methodology on which to draw when teaching clients. These are based on certain assumptions (except in the area of brain trauma) that the client understands the same concepts of body image, position in space, language, object recognition, sensation awareness and so on, as everyone else. None of these assumptions should be made with people who have learning difficulties if a successful outcome is to be achieved. They may be deprived of understanding not because of any intellectual deficit, but through lack of stimulation from physical contact, the inability to move and explore, an unstimulating environment and, sadly, the low expectations of others.

CASE STUDY 7

Pamela R

Ms R, a woman in her fifties, was being seen by a therapist in a hydrotherapy pool in the hospital. The therapist had little experience of people with learning difficulties, so advice was sought from a therapist in this field.

Hydrotherapy had been chosen as a medium to enable this woman, who was wheelchair dependent, unable to use her hands and non-verbally communicating, to gain some control of her body and a measure of independence.

When first seen in the pool Ms R was enjoying the sensation and was supported by four floats. The therapist felt this was a safe introduction to water. It was safe, but why, when someone has difficulty in learning, expect her to learn to do something twice, first with floats and then without them?

Floats prevented Ms R having to take any responsibility for herself, thus preventing her from experiencing the sensation of floating and learning about the buoyancy of the water. Apart from this, the floats disguised any movement she had. The therapist had been trying to help Ms R to move through the water and adjust her position. This had not been achieved.

Certain assumptions had been made which interfered with her learning of these skills.

1.   A full explanation had been given, but not using words and concepts that the client could understand. This does not mean that communication should be childish or patronising. On the contrary, it recognises that the client's experience in all aspects of living, including language, has been limited.

Communication is not only the expression of thoughts and ideas, but the interpretation of these thoughts and ideas by others, and in this case communication had not been as effective as expected.

2. It had been assumed that Ms R would need floats to feel safe. However, the same security can be given by correct physical support from the therapist and by adjusting the hold. The client should be given whatever amount of responsibility he or she is able to cope with. It is also better to enable the client to seek and accept independence in this way than to use floats which give a false sense of security and encourage an unrealistic expectation of abilities.

3. The assumption that Ms R had an awareness of her body and knew how to cause movement had also been made. This proved not to be true as Ms R, when tested, did not appreciate that if she lifted her head then her feet would lower in the water, and that turning her head would help her to roll over. This may seem difficult to believe, but if the client had always been lifted and moved without participating herself (because of either lack of time or ignorance of the time delay which people with learning difficulties have), how would she have learnt about cause and effect?

4. It was also assumed that Ms R would enjoy the sensation of standing in the pool, since the buoyancy of the water would make her feel lighter and easier to support. This assumption proved to be only partially true. She was thrilled to be upright for the first time in her life, but it is easy to forget the emotional trauma this can cause a client who has no verbal language with which to express her excitement, fear and joy – and her confusion as to why she had not done this before and whether she would be able to do it on land! Her only means of expression was to cry. The physiotherapist's reaction was to look for signs of physical pain.

This was a learning experience for all concerned as it took a week of careful communication on the part of the carers, speech therapist and physiotherapist to learn about these emotions. It must have been unbelievably frustrating and disappointing for her to try to share her joy with others who did not understand. In this case, who had the learning difficulty?

Once Ms R was approached with different cognition and attitudes she was able to progress. Ms R was given the reasons for the hydrotherapy course, and the aims and objectives to be accomplished in a language which she understood and appreciated. She was then given the option of continuing the therapy. Having indicated her wish to continue, a programme was devised to suit her.

Teaching occurs in all contact with clients. It must be consistent, and it should allow time for learning tasks, skills or behaviour. As Peto said, 'No time of day is better for learning than another'. Individuals have their own rate of learning and will often respond better to one particular technique or activity than another. They will always respond better to a person they like, so personality is important.

The assessment sets a baseline from which teaching begins. Teaching is carried out by explanation, instruction, example, practice, monitoring and sometimes, as an added incentive, inducement and reward.

Explanation

First ask the client, carer or advocate what problems they have with the skills they wish to learn; in the case of clients use whatever communication method they have to establish the problem. Tell the client what you wish to do, and why and how you are going to help. You should try to establish eye contact as part of the learning process, since the client will receive a better reaction and more willing communication from others if he or she can achieve this skill. Eye contact shows an awareness of others which enables communication to take place.

Insist also that the client listens to you while you explain in a simple and consistent way what you want to do. Task analysis technique should be used in some cases on language until the sentence is appropriate to the client's understanding.

For clients who are visually impaired or blind the approach must naturally be different as a sudden touch or unfamiliar voice can be both frightening and intrusive. It is surprising how familiar people are when touching blind people. Contact is not always welcome, and everyone is entitled to personal space.

For clients with a hearing impediment make sure that hearing aids are being worn if they are required. If the client is profoundly deaf, make sure you use Makaton signing or picture representation if it will facilitate easier communication with the client. The speech therapist can provide advice and assistance with this. The therapist should position him or herself in front of the client so that the client can see the physiotherapist's face and can then become involved. It is more difficult to begin communication with clients who are impaired in both sight and hearing. Here advice should be obtained from parents or carers who know the clients well and who could help in the introduction of the therapist.

The first thing is to try to establish a way in which the client can recognise the therapist, perhaps by a certain sign, by contact with something that the therapist constantly wears, or by smell (e.g. the therapist using the same perfume or aftershave). The therapist must be aware that a client will be fearful in any new situation when he or she has no reference point. The attitude associated with fear or anxiety can be mistaken for challenging behaviour, and this label can have detrimental effects on how the client is perceived and treated by others.

CASE STUDY 8

Gillian A

Ms A was a young woman of thirty, living in an institution. She was blind, had learning difficulties and was known to exhibit challenging behaviour. She spent most of her time crawling on her knees and finding her way around. She could stand and walk, but only on her toes, and her balance was erratic. She was often aggressive in her behaviour towards others, and when encouraged to help herself she would refuse by pushing, hitting and head-butting her carers.

She was referred to the physiotherapy department in the institution by a very concerned carer who advocated on her behalf. The carer insisted that Ms A needed the experience of getting out of her home environment, and that her behaviour resulted from boredom, lack of stimulation and fear. 'No one would try because she was so difficult' was the carer's opinion.

The therapist required a period of observation to get to know Ms A, and to allow her to get to know the therapist's voice. It took some time before Ms A would tolerate the therapist sitting beside her. After discussion with the clinical psychologist, the carers and another physiotherapist it was decided that two physiotherapists would be required. Ms A would then need to get to know the other physiotherapist, but only one therapist would give directions to Ms A so as to prevent confusion.

The therapists told Ms A what was to happen and what they hoped to achieve, and this was reinforced by the carers. The short-term goal was to get outside and walk along the corridor, a matter of 50 metres. The long-term goal was to get outside and walk to the shops or surrounding woods. Another long-term goal was to be able to get into a car and go for a drive, which was functional and would foster Ms A's independence.

The first session proved to be more strenuous than either therapist imagined. Ms A pushed, kicked, head-butted and refused to walk. She was encouraged, soothed and finally told that her behaviour was unacceptable, but that no matter how frightened she was it would be all right and she would get used to it.

After the first attempt the situation was reviewed by the therapists. Although exhausted from the effort, they decided that Ms A deserved perseverance on their part. The opportunity of widening horizons and possibly opening the way to a more fulfilling lifestyle should not be abandoned after one session. The ethics of the situation were discussed, and the multi-disciplinary team agreed that, even though early intervention was difficult for her, it was worthwhile continuing.

To provide continuity of contact and give Ms A time to learn, she was seen twice a week by the same therapists and a route established in order that she could familiarise herself with it and recognise where she was being taken. This took two months, during which time Ms A gradually accepted the therapists and struggled less when asked to go for a walk.

After three months Ms A walked with the therapists along the corridor for 150 metres with only a token head-butt. After four months stairs were introduced, which again caused aggression through fear, but the problem was talked through slowly, and eventually stairs too were accepted. Each new experience had to be introduced slowly in stages, with suitable explanations and support.

Within six months Ms A was walking with two therapists out of the home, along the corridors, up the stairs, across the grass and along a pavement on her way to the shops. At this stage one therapist was replaced, with careful introductions, by a physiotherapy helper. This caused less agitation than expected. Eventually Ms A and her carer went for trips alone. Ms A's balance improved, and when tired her habit of toe walking ceased. At this stage the whole process had to begin again when Ms A was introduced to a car.

Eventually introducing new experiences took less time and Ms A broadened her lifestyle considerably. Her challenging or complex behaviour encouraged the physiotherapists to bring all their experience and techniques to bear; to change the attitude of Ms A and also the attitudes of others towards her.

Instruction

One simple means of accomplishing a task is to tell the client what to do and how to do it. This can be very effective with many clients. If the client is blind then the therapist can use his or her own body to guide the client into the task to be accomplished, or facilitation can be used to get the client to achieve a task.

If a client has a hearing impairment then demonstration of the task is effective. For example, the therapist simply demonstrates the task in hand and the client can follow the therapist's example. It has to be noted that a client will react particularly well if he or she likes the therapist.

Practice

The only way to learn is by trying out the exercise, activity or leisure pursuit, and practising it many times so that proficiency is achieved. This practice should be monitored carefully, since it would be cruel and insensitive to allow a client to learn a task incorrectly and then have to re-learn the task correctly.

Incentive

This is a difficult area since the ethics are confusing. Bribery is wrong, but praise for an achievement is acceptable. Praise for a mediocre attempt, on the other hand, is patronising. To coin a phrase, 'The correct rate of pay for a job is acceptable, but token payment for a job well done is an insult.'

Before learning can be achieved the therapist must examine the tasks or skills to be learnt and break them down into component parts. Each part is taught separately so that the client can learn an element at a time, building up these competences one by one into a total task or skill.

Prompting is an action which can be done verbally, by touch or by both, and as soon as the client understands these prompts they can then be faded out and removed altogether.

CASE STUDY 9

David

David, a little boy of four in a 'special school', was working with his physiotherapist to gain control of his right arm and hand. He had cerebral palsy with athetoid movements, and was trying to place his hand on a musical keyboard in front of him.

This was a first step towards achieving the long-term goal of using his hand on a communication board. To afford David the best possible assistance he was seated in a position which controlled his body and allowed him to concentrate on his hand movements. Achieving the goal would take many months and would have to be seen by the four-year-old as a game. It would require considerable enthusiasm and ingenuity to keep this game alive so that David would want to play and enjoy doing so.

The order in which this was done was as follows:

1. *Demonstration and physical prompting.* To begin with the therapist held David's right arm and helped him to move it across his body in a proprioceptive neuromuscular facilitation (PNF) pattern on to the keyboard. When struck the keyboard made a musical sound which delighted him.

2. *Sensation.* David's arm was stroked and held to reinforce and facilitate the movement.

3. *Verbal prompting.* A simple sentence was used, not a barrage of complicated changeable sentences which would only have caused confusion. David understood clearly what 'Put your hand on the music' meant.

4. *Watching.* The therapist watched carefully for any movement, flicker of finger or even intent, and gave verbal reinforcement such as 'That's good David, I can see you are trying.'

5. *Time delay.* To begin with the therapist did not realise how long the time delay factor was between her request and the initiation of the movement by David. Once this was appreciated, David was allowed to react in his own time and proved to the therapist that he could move his arm. Often this delay is not appreciated and the therapist steps in too quickly, preventing any active movement and negating the effort made by the client. This can cause such frustration to the client that he or she will give up trying.

6. *Staging.* David was not expected to achieve the whole movement in one go. The therapist watched carefully to

see David's initial movement and with physical assistance helped him to finish the full range of movement in order to touch the keyboard and 'make music'. The therapist gradually withdrew the physical assistance at different stages of the movement as soon as David could manage them, until finally he could achieve the whole movement on his own.

As David progressed less physical prompting was necessary, less reinforcement was given, David's movements were more noticeable and he needed less encouragement. All he needed eventually was a verbal prompt and he would move his arm over and place it on the keyboard to make music.

From this learnt movement David was able to make choices on his own between two objects and even to touch and move a switch.

Preparation for teaching

When teaching theory or practical skills there needs to be adequate preparation, whether the teaching takes place in a one-to-one situation or in a lecture room full of students. It is important to give confidence to the people receiving the knowledge so that they are willing to accept these skills and, more importantly, to practise them. Preparation, presentation, demonstration and practice are all involved in this exchange of information, and will require different levels of attention depending on who is receiving the information and on the situation where this is taking place.

At one time or another we have all been on the receiving end of a bad or ill-prepared lecture, and we know the frustration this engenders. It is an insult to the intelligence of the audience and a waste of valuable time and resources. Each therapist has his or her own technique, but preparation is essential for all, whether it is to show someone how to help a person transfer from one chair to another, or to teach task analysis and goal planning to colleagues.

A prerequisite of preparation is to know the following:

Who is to be taught?
Where is this teaching to take place?
What style or approach should be adopted?
What will the environment be, and what environmental restraints are present?

What equipment or other resources are available?
What equipment might be required?
What documentation is required?

Time afforded to preparation is time well spent as it gives the physiotherapist confidence to know he or she is well prepared for the session and has everything necessary at hand. Then the physiotherapist can concentrate on the teaching itself. In fact, preparation prevents poor performance.

Preparation for teaching a client

What are the client's referred needs?
Where will the assessment take place? Is the venue relevant? Is it safe?
What equipment is necessary? Is it available? Does the equipment need to be transported to the client?
What documentation is required?
What assistance is necessary? For example, the client may be immobile requiring two people to begin rehabilitation or may challenge the therapist by their behaviour and assistance may be of help in these circumstances.

Preparation for teaching the carers

Explanations need to be prepared on the following:

Why it is necessary to help with the agreed programme
When should the carer help with the programme?
How should the carer help with the programme?
When should the carer not help? This advice is often the most difficult area to convey. It involves trying to understand the client's need for independence so that learning can take place.
What written information or instructions should there be on the programme to be followed?
What special equipment would make management easier? This may need to be found with the assistance of other disciplines, e.g. a hoist from occupational therapist.

What space is available for client, carer and physiotherapist to work together safely?

Preparation for lectures

What is the subject of the lecture to be?
How long is the talk to take?
What are the priorities?
Where is the venue to be?
What equipment is necessary? Is it available, or does it need to be transported?
What memory assistance is required? For example, if cue cards are required, these have to be used discreetly so as not to detract from the speaker. If lecture notes are used, make sure that a lectern or table is available so that hands are free to demonstrate a point or action.

Care is necessary when preparing cards or notes:

1. Always number each page in case they are moved or dropped: it's quicker to re-assemble them.
2. If acetates are part of the lecture, number or mark them and have that number in the correct position in the lecture notes, thus ensuring an easy flow from speech to visual display.
3. Devise a way to hold lecture notes together that facilitates easy, noiseless and efficient access to the notes.

Visual aids may be useful. Check to see what visual aids are available at the venue, inform them of your requirements or arrange to take your own. When using an overhead projector it is easier to cover the part of the acetate not yet required by putting the paper underneath the acetate. This prevents the distraction of the paper slipping. Remember, a good picture is worth a thousand words!

Make sure that you can be heard. If there is a microphone available, make sure that you know how to use it. Leave enough time before the lecture to try it out. Handouts, if required, should be carefully prepared, well-presented and left in an easily accessible place. Finally, make sure that drinking water is available.

Preparation for seminars

What is the course content and title? An interesting title should be chosen.

When is the seminar to take place? The date set must allow time to advertise the course and to receive replies and application forms. Advertising includes the design and printing of programmes.

Where is the venue to be?

Who are the speakers? Speakers should be arranged and confirmed by letter.

Have costing discussions been opened, and estimates for the provision of beverages and lunches been obtained and agreed? If the seminar is on 'alternative therapies', it is useful to bear in mind that herb or fruit tea might be more appropriate than caffeine-based drinks. The costs of the venue, speakers, food, equipment and travel should be taken into consideration before setting the cost to the participants.

Has a record been kept of all correspondence?

Has a list of course members been completed? Members should be sent programmes, location maps and any special enclosures, e.g. pre-course reading. Speakers should also be sent all necessary details.

Has the venue been informed of course members, the programme, any equipment necessary and special instructions, e.g. dietary preferences?

Have evaluation sheets been planned and prepared?

After the seminar the following actions are necessary:

1. The list of course participants should be filed.
2. Further information should be sent if this has been agreed.
3. Thank-you letters and expenses should be sent promptly to speakers.
4. Evaluation slips should be returned and analysed. Notes about how to improve the lecture should be made.
5. Accounts must be completed.

Presenting a lecture

When lecturing, poor appearance, stance and communication skills and nervous habits can all detract from the information exchange.

Appearance

The lecturer should be neat and tidy, and should wear clothes that do not distract from the talk to be given. The clothes should be appropriate for the task in hand and allow for comfortable active demonstration if this is to be part of the lecture. Rattling jewellery, unfastened buttons or untied laces will distract the audience from the content of the lecture and should be avoided.

Stance

It is important to decide whether to sit or stand when giving a lecture. Movement is distracting, so this must be taken into consideration when thinking about how to stand, where to stand and how to move about the floor or platform – a jack in the box is not easy to listen to. Remember also that it is important to see the audience and to be seen by them.

Communication

Firm friendly eye contact is necessary in order to receive attention and to gauge the reaction obtained from others. Speech should be clear, well-modulated, understandable and pitched at the correct level for the individual or group. Jargon, hesitation and hemming and hawing should be reduced to an absolute minimum.

Timing as well as volume is important to everyone, but especially to those with a hearing impairment. Time must also be allowed for viewing any visual display and for the audience to take notes if this is required. Gesture and Macketon signing should be used to assist verbal communication where this leads to more complete comprehension by the client or group.

Working with ethnic minorities where language may be a hindrance to communication, an interpreter should be employed.

(Languages may be a necessary addition to the physiotherapy curriculum in the future, in view of the development of the European Community and the establishment of a multicultural society).

Nervous habits

Nervousness is understandable and certain habits cannot be fully eradicated, but there are a variety of habits which can detract from or even ruin an otherwise excellent lecture. Continually straightening clothes, pushing hair out of the eyes, tapping with fingers or a pencil, and pulling one's ears at irritating intervals should all be avoided. Some people need to use their hands as an extension of their speech, but this has to be controlled to enhance the lecture rather than detracting from it. Watching oneself on a video recorder can be a salutary experience.

The venue

Lifting principles and handling can be taught in a lecture room, but lecturing alone is insufficient. It is necessary to monitor these procedures in the home environment with the client and carers to ensure the client's comfort and safety. Lifting should be eliminated as much as possible by the use of hoists where practicable and safe.

Student placements

In most areas of physiotherapy, initial contact about a student placement is made from the physiotherapy school, college or university. The service for people with learning difficulties is not always seen as the valuable placement it is, and representations should be made to the education establishments to encourage such placements.

Aims and objectives

The aim of student placements is to gain experience in the approach to, understanding of and management of people with learning difficulties. At the end of a placement students should be able to:

1. Apply relevant theoretical and practical skills previously learnt when working with clients.
2. Assess a client – remembering the SRV philosophy – and produce a programme plan based on personal strengths and needs.
3. Have an understanding of the task analysis approach to helping clients to achieve success.
4. Participate within the staff team and have an understanding of the role of each member of the multi-disciplinary team.
5. Keep accurate and legally correct written reports of all intervention undertaken.
6. Understand the policies on confidentiality and other essential organisational policies.

Pre-placement procedures

Discussion with the student establishment should take place to find out the following:

What are the aims, objectives and expectations of placement?
What is the time scale involved?
How many students are to be expected?
Which year are the students in?
What have they covered in the curriculum?
What teaching have they had on learning difficulty? If none, it would be helpful to negotiate lecture time to give an introduction into this field.
Who will monitor the placement?

Arrangements should be made for a tutor to visit the placement area.

Preparations for the placement

Discussion should take place with staff on areas of work, supervision, student programme, confidentiality, special district policies and balance of staff caseload. Other disciplines should be informed, and multi-disciplinary visits arranged in order to give the student added experience.

Training should be arranged if necessary, e.g. a clinical supervisor's course might be useful. Training allowances would then need to be organised.

The student placement must then be discussed with clients. It is necessary to seek permission from clients and, in the case of children, their carers to visit their homes if this is appropriate. It is also necessary apart from courteous to ask if they would have any objection to students learning to assess and work with them.

The student programme should be planned to include time for the following:

1. Introduction to service personnel.
2. Learning surroundings.
3. In-service training.
4. Reading, especially of important policy documents.
5. Visits to homes, team bases.
6. Assessing which clients the students will work with and which hydrotherapy units, leisure centres, riding establishments, etc. are to be visited.

A day-to-day work programme is essential if the placement is to last for only a week.

Letters should be sent to students in advance, including necessary information. For example, students should be told that a uniform is not worn in this service and that they may need special clothes such as a swimsuit, tough boots for hiking, etc. Students should be given the time of arrival, the location of the office or hospital, and a map of how to find it. Pre-placement reading should also be included.

A student package should be prepared so that students will have notes to refer to later. The package should be typed and stored for the students' arrival. An example of a student package is given in Figure 6.1.

STUDENT PACKAGE 1991

X HEALTH AUTHORITY

Physiotherapy staff

Superintendent physiotherapist:
Senior community physiotherapist:
Senior physiotherapist (X patch):
Physiotherapist:
Secretary:

Student programme

Monday	9.00	Staff meeting
	9.30	Introduction
		Social role valorisation
	10.30	Coffee
	10.45	Plan of action
	12.30	Lunch
	1.20	Lifting and handling
	2.45	Tea
	3.00	Wheelchairs and their adaptations
	4.00	Study time
Tuesday	9.30	Assessment
	10.30	Coffee
	10.45	Assessment continued
	12.30	Lunch
	1.20	Writing up assessment notes
	2.45	Tea
	3.00	'Annie's Coming Out' –
		video and discussion
Wednesday	9.30	Discussion and teach-in
		on the sensory-deprived
	10.30	Coffee
	10.45	Lecture on programme for
		individual needs (PIN)
	12.30	Lunch
	1.20	Afternoon in the community
Thursday	9.30	Programme planning
	10.30	Coffee
	10.45	Task analysis
	12.30	Lunch
	1.20	Afternoon of hydrotherapy
Friday	9.30	Study time
	10.00	Morning in the community
	12.30	Lunch
	1.20	Mobility techniques and facilitation
	2.45	Tea
	3.00	Feedback on week's activities

Rotational placements

One way of improving integration of people with learning difficulties into the generic service and of encouraging physiotherapists into this speciality is to introduce rotational placements. Rotational placements allow physiotherapists, especially those newly qualified, to work for set periods of time (usually four to six months) in different areas of physiotherapy, such as orthopaedics, neurology and paediatrics. In the last few years the service for people with learning difficulties has offered placements, but since physiotherapy for people with learning difficulties is still not seen as a particularly interesting speciality, it is essential that the placement should be well planned and successful. Placements are not easy to arrange when there are clients still living in institutions as well as clients living in the community.

The following information should be sent before placement:

1. Practical information, e.g. location.
2. Aims and objectives of placement.
3. Handouts covering policies, risk taking, etc.
4. Plan of induction.
5. Pre-rotation reading.
6. Names of staff personnel.

A typical timetable might include the following:

Week 1
1. Introduction to physiotherapy staff.
2. Familiarisation with department, institution or team base.
3. Understanding of departmental policies and procedures.
4. Introduction to area of work.

Week 2
1. Introduction to the client for whom the physiotherapist will be responsible.
2. Assessments to begin and assistance to be given as required.
3. Opportunties to watch seniors work and assess clients.
4. Introduction and teaching on programme for individual needs (PIN).
5. Visits to other departments for experience of multi-disciplinary working.

6. Lifting and handling sessions: there is a constant need for these to be taught to carers.

Week 3
1. Teaching on strengths and needs, programme planning and task analysis.
2. Time for writing notes and reading.
3. An early morning shift (if possible) to give the therapist an opportunity of seeing the problems from the carer's point of view.

Week 4
1. The physiotherapist, now more confident, continues with caseload.
2. An assessment to be written up and assistance given on planning task analysis and time scales.

Month 2
1. The physiotherapist continues with caseload and programme planning.
2. Opportunities taken to attend in-service training and other suitable courses, e.g. Makaton.

Month 3
1. The physiotherapist continues with caseload.
2. Visits with the team physiotherapist in the community to day centres, community homes and sports centres where therapists work (e.g. trampolining).

Month 4
1. The physiotherapist continues with caseload.
2. Visits to other services outside the district.
3. Caseload is handed over and feedback given on placement.
4. Check how the placement can be improved for next time.

Physiotherapists involved in this service often find it hard to understand why there is a fear of people who have learning difficulties; they rightly see the clients in the same way they see the rest of the population. However, this fear must be taken on board when students and new physiotherapists first enter this service, and dispelled through explanation, guidance and meeting the clients – who are their own best advocates.

Some clients are unpredictable and it takes a long time to get to know and understand them. It is therefore unrealistic to leave students unsupervised in this area of service, which is why student placement is so time consuming. However, if the clients are to be seen with respect and dignity in the community and acute physiotherapy services in the future, then placements are worth the commitment required and should be preserved.

Chapter 7

Multi-disciplinary working

Introduction

The term 'multi-disciplinary working' (MDW) means a practice whereby a group of professionals, specialising in a specific area of therapy, work together for the good of the client to provide a package of care suitable for each individual.

In theory, MDW is an excellent concept. However, many people unfortunately only pay lip service to the idea. In reality, it requires a great deal of thought, effort, communication, co-operation and care on the part of everyone to make it feasible, so that it can produce a cohesive, functioning and supportive team.

Working in a team

A team is not just a group of people sharing a team base; it is at best a group of people sharing a philosophy, setting goals, targets and using each other's knowledge in a constructive way for the overall benefit of the client. A team can consist of the following members:

Speech therapist
Clinical psychologist
Occupational therapist
Physiotherapist
Social worker
Administrator
Support manager
Patch manager

These usually work together at a team base, in close proximity to facilitate easy access to each other's skills and also to allow for immediate communication.

Some teams consist of a number of professionals with various responsibilities, who work at separate bases and come together for frequent meetings at a team base. The core team of a secretary, administrator, social worker and community worker is permanently based there. This is a less cohesive team, and extra effort with communication is necessary in this situation.

Belbin (1981) has made a long study of the best mix of characteristics in a team, and has formed a list of roles which are needed in order to achieve a fully effective group. He attributes the following titles to the personalities in the team: the chairman; the shaper; the plant; the monitor; the resource investigator; the organisational worker; the team worker; and the finisher. Whatever the names used to describe the members who contribute to the formation of a successful team, the characteristics required are the same:

1. There must be one person who presides over the team and co-ordinates its effort. He or she talks and listens well, is a good judge of people and of things, and is a person who works through others.
2. One is highly strung, outgoing and dominant. He or she is the task leader and in the absence of the co-ordinater would leap into that role. The person's strength lies in his or her drive and passion for the task.
3. One is introverted but intellectually dominant. He or she is the source of original ideas and proposals, being the most imaginative member of the team. However, this person can be careless in detail and can resent criticism.
4. One monitors and evaluates progress within the team, is also intelligent but has an analytical rather than a creative mind. His or her contribution is in the careful dissection of ideas and the ability to see the flaw in an argument. This person is dependable but can be tactless and cold.
5. The resourceful one is a popular member of the team: extrovert, sociable and relaxed, he or she brings new ideas and developments into the group. However, this person is not

original or a driver, and therefore needs a team to pick up his or her contributions.

6. The practical organisers are the people who turn ideas into manageable tasks; plans are their thing. They are methodical, trustworthy and efficient. They hold the team together by being supportive to others, listening, encouraging, harmonising and understanding. They are likeable and popular, but uncompetitive. They are the sort of people who are not noticed when they are there, but who are missed when they are absent.

7. Without the finisher the team might never meet its deadlines. This is the one who checks the details, worries about the time scales and chivies others with a sense of urgency.

Too many of one type of person means that the team lacks balance. A team would be fortunate, however, to have a full complement of such personalities. In a small team, therefore, one person may perform more than one role, and small stable groups often get by without a full set of roles.

It is also important to be aware of the fact that some members are ambitious, career orientated and constantly striving to provide a service for users which achieves the optimum philosophical statement of the service in which they work. This is an admirable but stressful goal, and such members need support.

MDW is an approach worth striving for. It benefits not only the people who require the service, but also the carers and team members. It provides a fount of easily accessible knowledge which can only enhance everyone's skills. Not only are their professional roles available, but their special interests and talents may also be used for the benefit of the client. Some team members are also musicians, dancers, trampoline coaches, mountain climbers and so on. The psychologist trampoline coach can assist the physiotherapist with rebound therapy; or the climber speech therapist might help in the preparation of activities for clients' outward-bound activity.

To work as a member of a multi-disciplinary team the physiotherapist needs to have an understanding of what the other disciplines are and do. He or she must be willing, enthusiastic, open-minded and prepared to co-operate with the other therapists for the clients' benefit. There is no place for professional jealousy.

At first the physiotherapist may find it bewildering or even threatening to be part of a team. Training in isolation does not foster an understanding of other professional roles. Most physiotherapy careers begin in hospitals where there is little exchange of ideas or communication between the disciplines, simply because different specialist departments are separated on different floors or even in different buildings. It is difficult to get a holistic approach to the person in this way, and more hospitals are becoming aware of the situation and trying to remedy this.

Once settled into a team it is stimulating to be within easy reach of other professionals, such as speech therapists, occupational therapists, psychologists and support workers. The physiotherapist must, however, be confident of his or her ability and be assertive on behalf of clients.

The team is a forum for discussion, evaluation and support, but it has to be said that working in a highly motivated, articulate group brings its own problems. There is a need to understand the dynamics of a team meeting, to be aware of hidden agendas, even to have skills in such things as chairing meetings and taking minutes. Training departments or in-service training modules can provide the chairing and minute taking which will assist the physiotherapists and add to their skills. A lack of understanding of each other's roles could result in a breakdown of team harmony. To gain this knowledge of other roles in-service training should occur. The role of the speech therapist, for example, should be explained, including the type of involvement that the speech therapist has with clients. It would also be helpful to know where and how people see joint working occurring with the other professionals on the team.

If all the professions had and used such opportunities to explain their roles to each other, conflicts over role definition would be limited. Each profession would also see the need for co-operation around programmes, so that each team member would be able to reinforce the programmes of others where possible. When working with a client, for example, the physiotherapist should use the Makaton signs that the speech therapist is teaching the client, or use the appropriate approach to a client that the clinical psychologist has prepared.

Benefits of team working

It is important to understand the purpose of a team. A team provides opportunities for the following:

1. Bringing together a set of skills, talents and responsibilities, and allocating a particular job to each team member.
2. Controlling the workload. Work can be organised and controlled by appropriate individuals who take responsibility for their area of work.
3. Problem solving and decision taking.
4. Programme planning.
5. Information processing, passing on decisions and information.
6. Co-ordinating and liaising about activities.
7. Negotiation and conflict resolution.
8. Monitoring previous decisions and giving feedback.

Responsibilities

When someone with learning difficulties is referred to a team, the appropriate professional will be asked to meet the client and to assess his or her needs. Should this referral turn out to be inappropriate when the professional meets the client, the latter is referred to another member of the team. For instance, if the client is referred to an occupational therapist and after a home visit the occupational therapist considers that the client's needs should be met by the physiotherapist, at the next meeting of the team this suggestion will be made and the physiotherapist will then take over the management of the client.

Caseload

At the team meetings the current workload of each professional can be discussed. It is at this forum that the physiotherapist can say that his or her workload has increased to the extent where no more referrals can be taken on for a period of time. Service deficiencies can also be made known at the meeting. Team prioritising is helpful when there is much work and the time and resources are limited.

Problem solving

There are often people with complex needs, some of which are quite difficult to meet. The team meeting is an opportunity to discuss these needs and to seek advice and help from the other members of the team. It may be that another professional can come up with a better solution which will work for the benefit of the client. No one profession has a monopoly on good ideas.

Programme planning

Each professional involved with a client assesses the client's needs and plans a programme that may be carried out by that professional with the client and carers, without any input from the other team members. The team should be informed of the involvement of that staff member.

On other occasions there may be five or more members of the team involved at the same time. This calls for careful liaison and one person to head up the programme so that, for instance, the client and carers are not overwhelmed by the number of professionals visiting their home. If possible a single programme for the client should be devised with all the therapists feeding into it. This is easier for the client and carers to follow, and it can be incorporated into the daily routine of the client.

Information processing

One of the most vital areas when working in a team is communication. Whether verbally or in written form, it is essential that all those involved with clients are informed of what intervention is going on in the clients' lives.

Client team case notes are one way in which to do this. Each professional involved with a client should keep a record of his or her intervention in the client's personal notes, and these should be clear, legal and follow the audit criteria of the profession. It helps if the notes are concise and easily distinguishable from others, e.g. the physiotherapist uses yellow paper, social workers use blue, etc.

Liaison and co-ordination

Liaison is a large part of the workload of every member of the team: liaison with parents, schools, day centres, colleges, hospitals, consultants, advocates and families. It may call for tact, sensitivity, persuasion, negotiation and assertion for and on behalf of the person with learning difficulties. This liaison can take the form of written communication, face-to-face meetings, home visits or telephone conversations. Each method calls for its own skills.

Good communication between members of the team is essential if colleagues' skills are to be used to achieve a better understanding of clients. For example, a clinical psychologist will have a better understanding of a client with challenging behaviour and could suggest methods of approach which the physiotherapist could use in working with the same client. Sharing a base helps to facilitate communication.

Negotiation and conflict resolution

Team work requires its own skills. Members need to trust each other, communicate about objectives and be aware of the hidden agendas which may be used to further someone's ambitions or change a previously agreed decision.

Tolerance is essential when working with many personalities, and each member needs to blend with the others to produce a well-structured and united team. Mutual respect should be the watchwords for team meetings, but respect also has to be earned.

Feedback

Feedback is a method of expressing one's thoughts, fears and grievances in an acceptable and constructive way for the benefit of all concerned. In behavioural terms, feedback is a way of increasing our awareness of ourselves and the effect our behaviour has on others. It gives the opportunity of modifying or changing our attitude and manner if necessary.

Working within a group or team can be stressful at times, and it is important to remember that when trying to find an appropriate form of feedback plain speaking may not be the most suitable. If possible, begin with a positive comment which can be seen to be encouraging, and then make any negative comments. It is important not to save all the negative points up and express them all at once like an explosion, as that will only have destructive results. One must always remember not to wreck people's confidence. A good working relationship is based on trust. It is important, therefore, to give praise when it is due and not to be afraid to criticise constructively when necessary. Both of these require skilful handling. It is as difficult for some people to accept compliments as it is for them to receive criticism, and one has to learn to take both in one's stride.

When it comes to feedback it is much easier to give than to receive. However, one has to be aware that one's own behaviour may cause problems within the team. Being on the receiving end of feedback can be quite uncomfortable, but it is important to listen to the feedback and not to reject it out of hand.

Feedback is of little use to anyone unless something good comes out of it. The team can and should be a supportive one; professionals who care for their clients should take time to care for each other.

CASE STUDY 10

Margaret P

Ms P was a young woman of twenty still living in a children's home and about to leave school in two months' time. She was wheelchair dependent with cerebral palsy, non-verbal communication and learning difficulty.

Ms P was referred to the team by the social worker for community housing, since a children's home was no longer considered suitable for the young adult. A discussion took place as to Ms P's strengths and needs as the social worker saw them. It was agreed that more information was required and that, as Ms P had physical disabilities, the physiotherapist should meet her and make a report to the team. The social worker would see Ms P's parents about the possibility of a move into the community house. The support worker on the team was to be involved in the house and would also be liaising with Ms P's present home.

The physiotherapist met Ms P with her school physiotherapist. During the discussion a careful observation of Ms P was made, but it would not have been appropriate or professional to assess Ms P at that venue or at that time, since she had only just met the new therapist. The school therapist gave a full report on the physiotherapy programme that Ms P had been receiving.

At the next team meeting the observations were shared.

1. Ms P was sitting in a very high, large, specially adapted wheelchair which would be difficult to manoeuvre around a small house and difficult for support workers to lift her out of. It was also unsightly and not age appropriate. It tended to be intrusive, the chair being more noticeable than the person, and all the straps to help Ms P maintain her position did nothing to enhance her body image and also prevented any movement occurring. All the above gave cause for concern, as well as the fact that the chair had been specially purchased and her parents were pleased with it.

2. Ms P had considerable spinal deformity, which would require special postural, comfortable seating.

3. Ms P was non-verbally communicating, but she made very loud noises when she wanted attention.

4. Advice would be required from the occupational therapist on Ms P's housing needs and the adaptations required. A joint visit to the home in which she was living was arranged between the occupational therapist and the physiotherapist in order to do a joint assessment.

5. The support worker had visited the home and was concerned about the difficulty Ms P was having in eating. He felt that the speech therapist could help in this area, and he anticipated that the new staff team in her future home would need training in the physical management of Ms P and in assisting her with eating. He was also concerned that Ms P was difficult at night and would scream, so he asked the psychologist to investigate this.

Just in the planning for Ms P's individual needs the multi-disciplinary team was involved in using the various skills of social worker, physiotherapist, support worker, occupational therapist, speech therapist and clinical psychologist, and in liaising with the school, the children's home and Ms P's parents.

Multi-disciplinary working has many advantages and some disadvantages. However, by working as a team it is possible to produce a harmonious body of professionals who deliver an excellent package of care and the desired outcomes for people with learning difficulties.

References

Belbin, R.M. (1981) *Management Teams*, London: Heinemann.

Useful addresses

A Chance to Grow (for brain injured children)
5034 Oliver Avenue North, Minneapolis, Minnesota 55430, USA

AGOR
Via Rancisvalle 70, 37136 Verona, Italy

Association for All Speech Impaired Children (AFASIC)
347 Central Markets, Smithfield, London EC1A 9NH

Australian Centre for Brain Injured Children (ACBIC)
52–54 Argyle Street, St Kilda 3182, Australia

Bobath Centre
5 Netherhall Gardens, London NW3 5RN

British Association of Occupational Therapists
20 Rede Place, London W2 4TU

College of Speech Therapists
Harold Poster House, 6 Lechmere Road, London NW2 5BU

Foundation for Conductive Education
University of Birmingham, PO Box 363, Birmingham B15 2TT

National Association for the Deaf/Blind and Rubella Handicapped
164 Cromwell Lane, Coventry CV4 8AP

People First London and Thames
c/o The People First Office
Oxford House, Derbyshire Street, London E2 6HG.

Peto Andreas Intezet
Kutvolgyi UT6, Budapest XII, Hungary H–1125

Royal National Institute for the Deaf
105 Gower Street, London WC1E 6AH

Spastic Society Central Assessment Service
16 Fitzroy Square, London W1P 5HQ

Further reading

Alaszewski, A. (1986) *Institutional Care and Mental Handicap*, London: Croom Helm.

Ayres, A. J. (1980) *Sensory Integration and Learning Disorders*, Los Angeles: Western Psychological Services.

Badenock, John (1986) 'Communication in medical practice', *Journal of the Royal Society of Medicine*.

Baily, Jocelyn (1990) 'Reflexology: A step in the right direction', *Practical Health*, August.

Barnes, J., Dennis, C., Barrell, A. and Jenkins, J. (1989) *Standards for Good Practice in Physiotherapy Services for People with a Mental Handicap*, London: Association of Chartered Physiotherapists in Mental Handicap.

Baroff, George S., *Mental Retardation: Nature, cause and management*, Washington: Hemisphere Publishing Corporation.

Behraman, Richard E. and Vaughan, Victor C. III (1983) *M D Nelson Textbook for Paediatrics*, Philadelphia: W. B. Saunders.

Belbin, R. M. (1981) *Management Teams*, London: Heinemann.

Berg, Joseph M. (1986) *Science and Service in Mental Retardation*, London: Methuen.

Bobath, B. (1971) *Abnormal Postural Reflex Activity Caused by Brain Lesions*, London: Heinemann.

Bobath, K. (1963) 'The prevention of mental retardation in patients with cerebral palsy', *Acta Paedopsychiatrica*, vol. 3, no. 4, pp. 141–54.

Bobath, K. (1966) *The Motor Deficit in Patients with Cerebral Palsy*, London: Heinemann.

Bobath, K. and B. (1975) *Motor Development in Different Types of Cerebral Palsy*, London: Heinemann.

Bone, M., Spain, B. and Fox, M. (1972) *Plans and Provision for Mental Handicap*, London: Allen & Unwin.

Brown, J. (1972) 'Ward 99', *Nursing Times*, February.

Bullock, Margaret I. (ed.) (1990) *Ergonomics: The physiotherapist in the workplace*, Edinburgh: Churchill Livingstone.

Bury, M. (1974) 'Life on Yellow Ward', *New Society*, May.

Callahan, Michael, A paper on the background, current status and future direction of the systematic instruction system known as try another way and of Marc Gould & Associates: Marc Gould & Associates, PO Box 6135, Syracuse, New York NY 13217.

Clarke, Ann M. and A. D. (1958) *Mental Deficiency: The changing outlook*, London: Methuen.

Clarke, David (1986) *Mentally Handicapped People Living and Learning*, London: Bailliere Tindall.

Cottom, P. and Scrutton, A., *Conductive Education: A system for overcoming motor disorder*, London: Croom Helm.

Cotton, E. (1981) *Conductive Education and Cerebral Palsy*, London: Spastics Society.

Cowling, A. G., Stanworth, M. I. K., Bennett, R. D., Curran, J. and Lyons, P. (1988) *Behavioural Sciences for Managers*, 2nd edn, London: Edward Arnold.

Craft, Michael (1979) *Tredgold's Mental Retardation*, London: Bailliere Tindall.

Craft, Michael and Ann (1978) *Sex and the Mentally Handicapped*, London: Routledge & Kegan Paul.

Crossley, Rosemary and McDonald, Anne (1980) *Annie's Coming Out*, London: Penguin.

Dolman, G., *What to Do About Your Brain Injured Child*, New York: Doubleday.

Finch, John D. (1984) *Aspects of Law Affecting the Paramedical Professions*, London: Faber & Faber.

Grand, Raghu N. and Hudson, Barbara L. (1978) *Current Themes in Psychiatry*, London: Macmillan.

Handy, Charles B. (1976) *Understanding Organisations*, London: Penguin.

Hari, M. and Akos, K. (1988) *Conductive Education*, trans. Neville Horton Smith and Joy Stevens, London: Routledge.

Heaton-Ward, W. A. (1975) *Mental Subnormality*, Bristol: Wright.

HMSO (1988) *Community Care: An agenda for action* (Griffiths Report), London: HMSO, ref. 0113211309.

HMSO (1989a) 'Caring for people: community care in the next decade and beyond', White Paper, London: HMSO, Cm849.

HMSO (1989b) 'Working for patients. The Health Service: caring for the 1990s', White Paper, London: HMSO, Cm555.

Hunter, Ian (1986) *Brain Injury: Tapping the potential within*, Bath: Ashgrove Press.

Jones, T and Prowle, M. (1987) *Health Service Finance*, London: Certified Accountants Education Trust.

Kiernan, Chris and Jones, Malcolm C. (1977) *Behavioural Assessment Battery*, Windsor: NFER-Nelson.

Korman, K. and Glennerster, H. (1990) *Hospital Closure: A political and economic study*, Milton Keynes: Open University Press.

Kugel, R. and Wolfensberger, W. (eds), *Changing Patterns in Residential Services for the Mentally Retarded*, Washington, DC: Government Printing Office, pp. 179–95.

Levitt, Sophy (1984) *Paediatric Developmental Therapy*, Oxford: Blackwell.

Lindsey, Mary (1989) *Dictionary of Mental Handicap*, London: Routledge.

Love, H. H. (1985) *Cognitive Counselling and Persons with Special Needs*, New York: Praeger.

Meyer, G. W. and Stott, R. G. (1985) 'Quality circles: Panacea or Pandora's Box?', *Organisational Dynamics*, Spring, pp. 34–50.

Mullins, Laurie J. (1989) *Management and Organizational Behaviour*, 2nd edn, London: Pitman.

Nirje, B. (1970) 'The normalization principle: implications and comments', *Journal of Mental Subnormality*, vol. 16, pp. 62–70.

O'Brien, John (1981) *Principles of Normalisation: A foundation for effective services*, London: Campaign for People with Mental Handicap. Adapted for CMH by A. Tyne.

O'Toole, R. (1972) 'New deal for mentally handicapped', *British Hospital Journal and Social Review*, 29 July.

Ownes, F. and Jones, Ron (1989) *Statistics*, London: Pitman.

Pelosi, Tony and Gleeson, Margaret (1988) *Illustrated Transfer Techniques for Disabled People*, Edinburgh: Churchill Livingstone.

Philpot, Terry (1990) 'Out of sight, out of mind', *Community Care*, 22 November.

Pilkington, T. (1967) 'The changing subnormality hospital', *British Hospital Journal and Social Service Review*, 3 February.

Presland, John L. (1982) *Paths to Mobility in 'Special Care'*, Kidderminster: British Institute of Mental Handicap.

Quality Assurance Working Party (1990) *Standards of Physiotherapy Practice*, London: Chartered Society of Physiotherapists.

Rushfirth, S. (1985) 'Community physiotherapy services for people with mental handicap', *Physiotherapy*, March, vol. 71, no. 3.

Salmon, Michael A. (1978) *Developmental Defects and Syndromes*, London: HM-M Publishers.

Scotson, L. (1985) *Dorian: A child of courage*, London: Collins.

Scrutton, D. (ed.) (1984) *Management of the Motor Disorders of Children with Cerebral Palsy*, Oxford: Blackwell.

Turnbull, George I. (1982) 'Some learning theory implications in neurological physiotherapy', *Physiotherapy*, February, vol. 68.

Vojta, V. (1962) 'Ontogeny of infantile spasticity', paper presented to the Neurological Society of CSSR, Prague.

Williams, P., Brown, J. and Jones, K. (1975) 'The back ward syndrome', *New Society*, 3 July.

Wolfensberger, W. (1972) *The Principle of Normalisation in Human Services*, Toronto: National Institute on Mental Retardation.

Wolfensberger, W. and Glenn, L. (1973) *Program Analysis of Service Systems (PASS): A method for the quantitative evaluation of human services*, Field Manual, Toronto: National Institute on Mental Retardation.

Woolf, A. D. (1989) 'Osteoporosis: A preventable problem', *Care of the Elderly*, October, vol. 1, no. 5.

Yeates, Sybil (1980) *The Development of Hearing*, Lancaster: MTP Press Ltd.

Yule, William and Carr, Janet (1980) *Behaviour Modification for the Mentally Handicapped*, London: Croom Helm.

Index

Alaszewski, A., 5
Alzheimer's disease, 37, 84
anoxia, 19
Ashkenazy community, 19
assessment, 45–63
asylum, 4
ataxia, 20
athetoid cerebral palsy, 20
audit, 72

Bobath, B., 26, 32
Bobath, K., 26, 32
Bobath technique, 65–7, 79–80
Bone et al., 5
Brain-Stem Evoked Response, 53
Bury, M., 7

cerebral palsy, 20
chromosomal abnormalities,
    16–18
communication, 53–5
conductive education, 67, 81
cri du chat, 17
Crossman, R., 8

Derby mould, 62
Delacarto, C., 26, 80
development team, 9
diplegia, 20
Dolman, G., 26, 80
Down's syndrome, 16

Education (Handicapped
    Children) Act 1970, 24, 29
Educationally Subnormal (ESN),
    24
EEC Manual Handling of Loads
    Directive, 70
ENCOR, 10
environmental factors, 19–20
epilepsy, 22–3

galactosaemia, 18
Glenn, L., 2
Griffiths Report 1988, 12

hospitals
    Darenth Park, 10, 11
    Ely, 6
    Fieldhead, 9, 26
    Gogarburn, 26
    Harperbury, 26
    Leavesden, 8, 26
    Newchurch, 26
    Northgate, 8

infections, 20–1
institutions
    Park House, 4
    Starcross, 4

Kabat, H., 80